The Patient–Doctor Consultation in Primary Care

The Patient–Doctor Consultation in Primary Care
Theory and Practice

Jill Thistlethwaite
Penny Morris

ROYAL COLLEGE OF GENERAL PRACTITIONERS

LONDON · 2006

The Royal College of General Practitioners was founded
in 1952 with this object:

*'To encourage, foster and maintain the highest possible standards
in general practice and for that purpose to take or join with others
in taking steps consistent with the charitable nature of that object
which may assist towards the same.'*

Among its responsibilities under its Royal Charter the College
is entitled to:
*'Diffuse information on all matters affecting general practice and
issue such publications as may assist the object of the College.'*

British Library Cataloguing-in-Publication Data
A catalogue record for this book is available from the British Library

© The Royal College of General Practitioners, 2006
Published by the Royal College of General Practitioners 2006
14 Princes Gate | Hyde Park | London sw7 1PU

Designed and typeset at the Typographic Design Unit

Printed by Bell & Bain Ltd, Glasgow

Indexed by Carol Ball

ISBN 978-0-85084-307-1

Contents

Acknowledgements   *vi*

List of authors   *vii*

List of abbreviations   *viii*

CHAPTER 1
Introduction   1

CHAPTER 2
Consultation models: history and histories   15

CHAPTER 3
Shared decision making and patient partnership: involving patients
in management   35

CHAPTER 4
Sharing information: evidence and risks   55

CHAPTER 5
Consultation skills techniques and strategies in more depth   77

CHAPTER 6
Issues relating to changes in general practice affecting the
doctor–patient relationship   105

CHAPTER 7
Preparing for patients in the 21st century: learning to listen
and to engage   125

CHAPTER 8
Assessment of communication/consultation skills and competence:
what do we do and how do we do it?   147

CHAPTER 9
The patient voice in doctors' learning   175

CHAPTER 10
Electronic communication and issues relating to the consultation   205

CHAPTER 11
The consultation in the 21st century   223

Index   237

Acknowledgements

We would like to thank all the people we have worked with and learned from in Leeds, Manchester, London and Cambridge, especially the real and simulated patients who have helped us understand more about consultations.

Authors

Jill Thistlethwaite BSc MB BS PhD MMEd FRCGP FRACGP DRCOG is Associate Professor of Medical Education and Director of Research, Learning and Teaching in CIPHER (Centre for Innovation in Professional Health Education and Research) at the University of Sydney, where she also works as a GP at the University Health Centre. She is Chair of the prevocational education sub-committee of the Royal Australian College of General Practitioners. She moved to Australia from the UK in 2003. Prior to this she was Senior Lecturer in Community-Based Education at Leeds University Medical School, and a GP in West Yorkshire.

Penny Morris BA is Senior Lecturer in Communication Skills in the Medical Education Unit at the University of Leeds School of Medicine, UK, and is an associate director for the 'Fresh Start' programme at the London Deanery Postgraduate Department of GP Education and Training. She undertook a Harkness Fellowship to the USA to investigate the patient voice in health care and was on the taskforce for the conference 'Where's the patient's voice in health professional education?' in Vancouver in 2005. She has previously worked at Manchester and Cambridge universities, and with doctors, nurses and patients in the community.

David Topps MB ChB MRCGP FCFP CCFP is Associate Professor and Director of eLearning at the recently founded Northern Ontario School of Medicine (NOSM), Canada. Previously he was Assistant Professor in the Department of Family Medicine at the University of Calgary. He did his GP vocational training in Aberdeen, Scotland.

Abbreviations

CMFS	chronic multiple functional somatic symptoms
CQI	consultation quality index
DEN	doctor's educational needs
DIPEx	database of patient experiences of health and illness
DNA	did not attend
DNR	do not resuscitate
DoH	Department of Health
EBM	evidence-based medicine
GMC	General Medical Council
HRT	hormone replacement therapy
IBS	irritable bowel syndrome
ICEE	ideas, concerns, effect, expectations
IHD	ischaemic heart disease
ISDM	informed shared decision making
LAP	the Leicester assessment package
NPCRDC	National Primary Care Research and Development Centre
OPTION	observing patient involvement instrument
OSCE	objective structured clinical examination
OSLER	objective structured long examination record
OTC	over the counter
PDA	personal digital assistant
PDP	personal development plan
PEI	the patient enablement instrument
PMETB	Postgraduate Medical Education and Training Board
PMT	premenstrual tension
PPD	Personal and Professional Development
PRHO	pre-registration house officer
PUN	patient's unmet need
QoF	Quality and Outcomes Framework
RCGP	Royal College of General Practitioners
RPSGB	Royal Pharmaceutical Society of Great Britain
SHO	senior house officer
SMS	Short Message System
SP	simulated patient
TLA	three letter abbreviations
WHO	World Health Organization
WONCA	World Organization of Family Doctors

Introduction

This chapter explores:

● why another consultation skills book is needed ● evidence
of why communication skills still need improving ● standards
set by the General Medical Council (GMC) and the Royal College
of General Practitioners (RCGP) ● the RCGP curriculum relating
to consultation skills ● the outline of the book.

'Open your ears, doctor. Why do GPs fail to spot cancer? All
too often it's because they don't listen.'

Sᴏᴘʜɪᴇ Pᴇᴛɪᴛ-Zᴇᴍᴀɴ[1]

'The consultation is at the heart of general practice. It is the
central setting through which primary care is delivered. ...
The general practitioner who lacks a clear understanding of
what the consultation is, and how the successful consultation is achieved, will fail his or her patients.'

RCGP Cᴜʀʀɪᴄᴜʟᴜᴍ Sᴛᴀᴛᴇᴍᴇɴᴛ Nᴏ.2 – Tʜᴇ Gᴇɴᴇʀᴀʟ Pʀᴀᴄᴛɪᴄᴇ Cᴏɴꜱᴜʟᴛᴀᴛɪᴏɴ[2]

Two people have written the main part of this book: an academic general
practitioner who still works in general practice for part of the week (JT) and
a teacher and researcher in medical communication (PM). When we write
as 'we' our opinions relate to both these positions. When we write as 'I' the
views are related to our personal experience; which 'I' is which should be
apparent from the context. Our experiences relate mainly to primary care
in the United Kingdom but we do make reference to general practice in
other English-speaking countries. We also refer to our work in Australia
and the United States of America, while the author of Chapter 10 practises
in Canada.

The text is aimed foremost at practising general practitioners but we hope
that other health professionals who interact with patients will find it helpful.
It is also a useful resource for anyone involved in medical education, particularly those new to the field.

A general practitioner's personal journey (JT)

Like many doctors of my generation I went through medical school without any specific training in talking to, let alone listening to, patients. Indeed, I didn't meet a patient until halfway through my undergraduate course. After three years and just prior to finally getting onto the wards, we medical students were given a few hours of teaching on how to take a history and a couple of days on physical examination. Before my final examinations I was rarely formally observed talking to patients and certainly received little in the way of feedback about my skills. The aim of any interaction with a patient was to take a comprehensive history along set lines and to generate a differential diagnosis list. Students were asked about management plans, but certainly we never discussed these with the sick people we encountered.

Yet in my first year as a house officer I was expected to inform a family of the unexpected death of their mother after a routine operation. This was inappropriate for both the relatives and me.

In 1984 I was a GP trainee in the Chilterns. One half-day release session was run by David Pendleton, fresh from the publication of his co-authored book *The Consultation*.[3] (This book became a classic of general practice literature. It formulated an approach to the consultation that drew together in a practical and informative way the evidence for good communication, and defined a blueprint for the way GPs could work effectively with patients.) We spent the afternoon looking at videotapes (which were black and white, poor quality and very amateur) of our consultations and plotting consultation maps. David and the course organiser encouraged us to reflect on our communication and interpersonal skills. How we squirmed in embarrassment at the cues we had obviously missed from patients. Our ignorance of body language and use of jargon was all too apparent on the tapes. We were then introduced to the idea of asking patients about their ideas and concerns. I had possibly done this in a simplistic way before, but usually had only engaged patients in discussing such issues if they had volunteered anxieties without prompting. The suggestion was scary but exciting. However, I wasn't really sure what to do with the issues raised by such questioning. Too many years of hospital training had left me, a female, with a paternalistic viewpoint. If a patient was anxious at the start of a consultation, my careful questioning, diagnosis and subsequent management plan would allay any concerns. In the second part of the consultation the patient would rarely be able to utter a sentence except in acquiescence to my treatment decision. When it came to management it was usually a case of advising the patient what to do and prescribing drugs that I expected them to take without question. Advising isn't perhaps the correct word for every consultation. There was certainly an element involved of 'telling' the patient.

My own communication skills were learnt primarily 'on the job'. For the first decade of practice as a full-time GP I saw a patient every seven minutes. In the early years the consultation usually consisted of a focused history and a one-sided decision on treatment. Over time I began to explore patients' ideas, as this began to seem appropriate. Moreover, by seeing many of the same patients on a regular basis I was able to understand more fully patients' anxieties and their reasons for choosing whether or not to listen to my advice. The social context of people's lives also became important, as I realised that there were more to physical symptoms and unhappiness than disease.

Once I was a GP trainer and began to help my own trainees develop consultation skills by watching their videotapes and recording my tutorials, my own skills improved markedly. Seven minutes was no longer enough for a patient and, indeed, my practice partners eventually decided that consultations would last ten minutes.

○ **Simulated patient** *a person who has been trained to simulate an actual person accurately, including history, body language and emotional and personal characteristics.*

I continue to learn and improve. The concept of informed shared decision making seems a logical progression. Simulated patients (SPs) and expert patients have been important factors in my development. However, there are always new challenges that require new ways of working and communicating. The telephone and email consultation are facts of medical life. Many patients are highly knowledgeable about medical matters through the media and internet. People expect to be involved in decisions about their health care and to have frank discussions about risk and adverse reactions.

A medical educator's personal journey (PM)

When I was working with a group of young people who, like me, wanted to change the world I was asked to help doctors relate better to patients. I wasn't very interested at the time and didn't realise what a difference such work could make.

The first member of my family to go to college, I had gone to York University to study English and philosophy. I had always enjoyed acting. It was the late 1960s and at university I became involved with new forms of theatre.

One of these was a community action theatre group called Inroads, which a group of us formed to work on council housing estates with local people and their children. In 1972, we moved over the Pennines to Salford in Lancashire where the local authority, having heard of our work, offered us several streets of condemned houses in Lower Broughton, the 'Classic Slum', in which to live and work at a token rent. It was a period of great social change: the slums were being cleared and the brave new world of high-rise living was being promoted as a solution for extreme social deprivation. At this time, we began to respond to requests from the children's parents to produce material about their own lives, including rent rises and the state of the local hospitals.

Eventually, we became North West Spanner.[4] Members of the group moved on, and my partner and I shifted our base to the hills outside Manchester. For a while we worked in our local hospital as auxiliary and porter, sharing the power of patients' stories. In 1975, the Arts Council offered grants for experimental theatre and we were invited to apply. We won a grant to make a play about the closing of the mills that surrounded us. Our venues became factory canteens, working men's clubs and community centres.

During this time, we met Peter Barnet, a dedicated community worker whose best friend turned out to be the next Professor of General Practice at Manchester University, David Metcalfe. I had taken part in a role-play with Peter for community worker training, playing a woman talking about her problem child. David asked if we could develop similar training for student doctors.

Eventually, we were persuaded to give the work a try and became fascinated by the rich intensity of the role-played consultations. We felt that offering the story and voice of the patient for the community's future doctors could be useful. We developed this teaching with the department and beyond, as described further in Chapter 7.

I eventually moved on, in 1986, with a brief to innovate new teaching at Cambridge. Here, on the basis of the Manchester experience, I was able to develop an approach to communication learning that arose from the patient's perspective, rather than doctors' needs to manage patients. I have continued and developed this work, currently at Leeds University, which has been a centre of excellence for the involvement of patients and the community. Over the last 20 years, the work has involved researching, in collaboration with others, new ways to enable health professionals and patients to rethink old attitudes and approaches. It has involved work with students and their clinical teachers at Cambridge; with GPs, mainly in London; and with students, clinicians and patients at Leeds. Other 'Spanners' have moved on, too, but are still in healthcare training, and have been part of all of this work.

We also spent a significant year in Chicago, investigating the patient voice in health care, going back to our roots in community development. Here was a 14-year-old African American boy who had trained to be a 'patient teacher' in sessions run for medical students in his school by the community. He explained what he thought his role was in helping a medical student: 'It's not for me to *tell* her … it's for her to catch on.' He understood about empowerment for himself and those around him. He was part of the self-declared Westside Health Authority, led by Jackie Reed, where people's capacities and gifts are emphasised, not their deficits.[5]

Many years after the theatre group days, I was observing medical students talking to simulated patients during examinations at Leeds University. As in most UK medical schools at the time, these students had been exposed to two models of interviewing patients, one that entailed the classic taking of histories and the other that included eliciting the patient's view and experience of the problem. During the parts of the examination labelled as 'communication skills', many students added 'What are you worried about?' or 'Do you have any concerns?' in much the same way that they surveyed for other symptoms, and with as much engagement. They did not appear to know what these questions were for. It seemed their understanding of the role of the patient's view and experience in the medical conversation was that these were either feelings that the doctor could sort out, or wayward ideas that the doctor should sort out. This is an ongoing challenge for the field.

We have growing evidence that the key to improved health outcomes is increased participation in the consultation and health care.[6] Perhaps with the joint learning we touch on in Chapter 7, more students and doctors will be convinced of the capabilities of the Chicago school student and the need to engage with people like him.

Communication skills: can still do better

The patient-centred approach and patient partnership are now common terms. Vocationally trained GPs at least know about the concepts and may apply the skills in some consultations. Communication skills training takes place at both undergraduate and postgraduate levels because medical educators now widely recognise that failure of communication (both doctor–patient and between health professionals) is a major factor in adverse clinical events and poor patient outcomes. Two Australian studies in the 1990s found that communication errors were the leading cause of in-patient deaths, twice as common as inadequate clinical skills,[7] while half of all adverse events in general practice were associated with poor communication of some kind.[7,8]

Yet in spite of this increasing emphasis on communication and consultation skills training, newspapers and magazines are full of anecdotes about misunderstandings between doctor and patient. Patients complain that doctors don't listen, or that doctors are rushed and don't take time to explain. Many GPs are used to being asked by their patients to decipher the management strategies of their hospital colleagues. But GPs themselves are criticised for communication breakdowns and certainly we would all admit we could often do better. General practice and primary care have changed. There are ever-increasing demands on doctors to meet certain targets and to save money by prescribing fewer drugs, making fewer referrals and dealing with more healthcare problems and screening in primary care. Litigation is on the increase. This last situation serves to highlight even more the importance of communication, as suing the healthcare professionals often relates to a failure of communication between doctor, healthcare team, patient and family. These issues and the evidence for them will be discussed in the chapters that follow.

As will be mentioned in Chapter 3, the 2002 Commonwealth Health Fund International Health Policy Survey of Sicker Adults found that about 50 per cent of patients in the five countries surveyed, including the UK, felt that their regular doctor did not ask for their ideas and opinions about treatment and care.[9] A European survey found similar figures in that only 50 per cent of respondents felt their doctors listened carefully to them and gave a clear explanation of their problems and treatment; the British and Swiss doctors, however, were rated the highest for interpersonal skills.[10] A major factor explaining the low ratings in Europe generally is lack of training. With the trend towards shared decision making, doctors require skills in negotiation and explanation, discussion of risk and the ability not to sway patient choice due to their own beliefs and prejudices. This is important because 74 per cent of the European patients expected to be actively involved in treatment decisions.[10]

There are of course a number of books on communication skills and these will be acknowledged in this text. So why another book? We would answer that question by asking another: why is communication still a problem with all these helpful guides around? One issue is obviously the difficulty of putting theory into practice. There are many constraints to practising patient-centred care and even more in involving patients in decision making. On a day when all appointments are full, one partner is off sick and there is an upsurge in viral infections, communication can be reduced to its most basic form of a quick history and an even quicker pronouncement of the 'virus – antibiotics no use' mantra.

This book acknowledges these pressures and concentrates on communication within the general practice consultation and its aftermath. It does not offer easy solutions but takes another look at the consultation and doctor–patient interactions in a new century. The evidence is sifted and ways of working are suggested. We discuss the outcomes of poor communication such as low patient satisfaction and lack of adherence to treatment regimes.

This is not a how-to manual though there are lists and examples of strategies to improve communication. It complements other texts on communication and refers to these where relevant.

Another issue is a deeper one: are the ways that communication and consultation skills have been taught and learned missing something? The book also explores what patients and other voices in our communities offer for a vision of the 21st century consultation.

Setting standards

The GMC (General Medical Council) in *Good Medical Practice* [11] and the RCGP in *Good Medical Practice for General Practitioners* [12] list and discuss the attributes they consider to be important in doctors. Many of these are related to consultation skills (Box 1.1).

There are of course other components of communication and barriers to excellence, and these will be discussed in detail.

In 2004 the RCGP developed its six domains of core competencies, based on the 2002 WONCA (World Organization of Family Doctors) definition of the discipline of general practice. [13] The second domain is 'person-centred care' and the sixth is 'a holistic approach', which are both fundamental

---

Box 1.1 ○ **Good medical practice**

○ Treat every patient politely and considerately.

○ Respect patients' dignity and privacy.

○ Listen to patients and respect their views.

○ Give patients information in a way they can understand.

○ Give patients the information they ask for or need about their condition.

○ Respect the rights of patients to be fully involved in decisions about their care.

○ Excellent GPs respect the right of patients to refuse treatment or tests.

concepts linked to the consultation and communication skills. (The other domains are: 1) primary care management; 3) specific problem-solving skills; 4) a comprehensive approach; and 5) community orientation.)

New curriculum for general practice training

The new Postgraduate Medical Education and Training Board (PMETB) asked the RCGP to produce a new curriculum for general practice training. The new curriculum for general practice will come into force from August 2007. The curriculum, specified within a framework for a structured education programme, is designed to address the wide-ranging knowledge, competences, clinical and communication skills, and professional attitudes considered appropriate for a doctor intending to undertake practice in the contemporary UK National Health Service. It has been designed to inform the period of postgraduate medical education and training for general practice leading to the award of a Certificate of Completion of Training. This in turn will give the successful doctor eligibility for entry onto the General Medical Council's General Practitioner Register.[14]

The curriculum statement on the consultation includes the following:[2]

- demonstrate an understanding of the context in which the consultation happens

- demonstrate an understanding of the structure of the consultation

- demonstrate awareness that good consultation requires good professional attitudes (this includes ethics, reflective practice and recognising one's own limits).

There are learning outcomes specifically related to the consultation. They relate to what a GP registrar must be able to do at the end of general practice training, and are therefore the competencies expected of a qualified and certified GP. We will now consider the relevant learning outcomes and where they will be discussed in this book. The chapter is given after each item. If no chapter is given this is because the item is covered in different aspects throughout the text.

Demonstrate an understanding of the context in which the consultation happens
With *patients* this means:

- recognising that patients are diverse, that their behaviour and attitudes vary, e.g. by age, gender, ethnicity, social background and as individuals (Chapters 2, 6 and 9)

- responding flexibly to the needs and expectations of different individuals

- understanding the process by which patients decide to consult and how this can affect consulting outcomes

- recognising the GP's role and responsibilities towards the patient

- negotiating a shared understanding of the problem and its management with the patient, so they are empowered to look after their own health (Chapter 3)

- demonstrating commitment to health promotion while recognising the potential tension between this role and the patient's own agenda

- managing the potential conflicts between personal health needs, evidence-based practice and public health responsibilities (Chapter 4).

With the *patient's relatives, friends and supporters* this means:

- recognising that episodes of illness may affect more than the patient

- understanding the patient's right to confidentiality

- negotiating whether and how relatives might be involved.

With other *professional colleagues* this means:

- working successfully as a member of the primary care team

- working successfully with colleagues in secondary care and elsewhere

- working successfully with a range of other professionals such as Social Services.

In all cases this means recognising that 'working successfully' involves:

- understanding the role of professional colleagues and where their expertise lies

- drawing on this expertise as appropriate

- treating colleagues with consideration and respect

- understanding interprofessional boundaries with regard to clinical responsibility and confidentiality.

Demonstrate an understanding of the structure of the consultation

- Demonstrate familiarity with the common models of the consultation and how these models can be used to reflect on previous consultations in order to shape future consulting behaviour (Chapters 2 and 3).

- Demonstrate therefore in consultation performance:

  - an awareness that consultations have a clinical, psychological and social component, with the relevance of each component varying from consultation to consultation (Chapter 2)

  - an ability to deploy successfully the characteristics represented by the MRCGP examination (Chapter 8)

  - an ability to use techniques to limit consultation length when appropriate.

- Recognise that achieving a successful overall structure involves appropriate use of communication skills and therefore:

  - demonstrate in consultation an appropriate use of the skills typically associated with good doctor–patient communication (Chapters 2–6)

  - demonstrate in consultation performance an ability to adapt communication skills to meet patient needs (Chapters 2–6)

  - demonstrate the ability to formulate appropriate diagnoses, rule out serious illness and manage clinical uncertainty

  - demonstrate effective use of patient records (electronic or paper) during the consultation to facilitate high-quality patient care (Chapters 10 and 11)

  - demonstrate effective use of time and resources

  - understand how consultations conducted via remote media (telephone and email) differ from face-to-face consultations, and demonstrate skills that can compensate for these differences (Chapters 10 and 11).

Demonstrate awareness that good consultation requires
good professional attitudes

- Demonstrate familiarity with basic concepts in medical ethics.

- Demonstrate an ability to reflect on how particular clinical decisions have been informed by these concepts.

- Understand the need to share information with patients in an honest and unbiased manner (Chapters 3–5).

- Demonstrate ethically sound practice in consultation performance.

- Show an understanding of the importance of good professional behaviour and how it is manifest in successful consultations by:

  o demonstrating respect for patients, colleagues and others

  o demonstrating good team-working skills

  o keeping accurate, legible and contemporaneous records (Chapters 10 and 11)

  o making timely and appropriate referral

  o displaying good time-keeping.

- Demonstrate an understanding of the importance of reflective practice for good consultation technique by:

  o recognising the limits of one's own abilities and expertise (Chapters 4, 7 and 9)

  o undertaking self-appraisal through such things as reflective logs and video recordings (Chapters 7, 8 and 11)

  o recognising, monitoring and managing personal emotions arising from the consultation (Chapters 5, 7 and 9)

  o recognising how personal emotions, lifestyle and ill-health can affect consultation performance (Chapters 5 and 7).

Outline of the book

After this general introduction each chapter may be read as a stand-alone text. However, the chapters are complementary and build concepts, issues, problems and strategies towards the final chapter.

Chapter 2 concentrates on the medical history and information gathering and sharing. It gives an account of the medical history and how it is taken – or rather how it is elicited. Having a sense of the profession's history is important and shows how ideas are cyclical. Doctors were patient centred in some respects in the past, certainly towards their rich clients. Paternalism then became the way to work as the biomedical model gained ascendancy.

Today we are once again advised to adopt a patient-centred approach. This approach leads on to the concepts of patient partnership and shared decision making, which are dissected in Chapter 3. This chapter also looks at informed consent. Just what should GPs be telling patients and how do we know that patients want to be involved in decisions about their own health care? The balance between giving patients what doctors think they need and what *they* think they need is discussed.

Chapter 4 looks more closely at the type of information that patients require and ask for in order to make healthcare decisions. We discuss ways to describe risk and how to deal with uncertainty. Decision aids are likely to become more helpful in this process as more are developed and evaluated.

Some of the communication skills mentioned in earlier chapters are expounded in more depth in Chapter 5. We describe strategies for dealing with certain types of consultations and a variety of situations including breaking bad news, helping the frequent attender and coping with aggression. The references will be useful if you want to read more on these topics.

The changing nature of society and how this impinges on the consultation and the doctor–patient relationship is the topic of Chapter 6. How do we measure the quality of a consultation? Is continuity of care still possible or necessary? We recognise the diverse nature of some patient populations and that we may need to consult with an interpreter or advocate present.

Chapter 7 explores the development of communication and consultation skills training and ways of facilitating doctors to develop their perceptions and enhance their skills.

Chapter 8 looks at how communication and consultation skills are assessed, and at some of the science behind assessment. We explore the difference between competence and performance. Revalidation and methods of demonstrating performance are discussed. There is information on the membership examination for the RCGP and other assessments.

Chapter 9 explores the contribution of the patient voice to new understandings of the consultation. We examine the changing role of patients in learning and how to ensure the patient voice is heard, including within lay teachers such as SPs. We recognise the importance of the voice of the person within the professional, too. We discuss the implications for doctors and for patients.

Chapter 10 recognises the information technology revolution, the e-consultation and the rise of the computer in the consulting room. David Topps is a British-trained GP now working as an academic in Ontario, Canada. He has substantial experience in the electronic dimensions of the consultation and explores the benefits and problems arising from changes in communication brought about by scientific advances.

The final chapter pulls things together and runs through a present-day consultation, its preparation and aftermath. This includes record keeping and professional development.

REFERENCES

1 Petit-Zeman S. Open your ears doctor. The *Guardian*. 3 February 2004, p. 16.

2 www.rcgp.org.uk/pdf/educ_curr2%20The%20GP%20Consultation%20Jan%2006.pdf (RCGP Curriculum Statement No.2 – The General Practice Consultation) [accessed May 2006].

3 Pendleton D, Schofield T, Tate P and Havelock P. *The Consultation: An Approach to Learning and Teaching*. Oxford: Oxford University Press, 1984.

4 Dalton E. Big in Dudley: the story of North West Spanner. *North West Labour History Journal* December 2002; **27**: 68–74.

5 Morris P. Citizens in health care. In: Hambleton R and Taylor M (eds). *People in Cities: A Transatlantic Policy Exchange*. Bristol: SAUS Publications, 1992, pp. 214–34.

6 Michie S, Miles J and Weinman J. Patient-centredness in chronic illness: what is it and what does it matter? *Patient Education and Counseling* 2004; **51**: 197–206.

7 Wilson R M, Runciman W B, Gibberd R W, *et al*. The Quality in Australian Health Care Study. *Medical Journal of Australia* 1995; **163**: 458–71.

8 Bhasal A L, Miller G C, Reid S E, *et al*. Analysing potential harm in Australian general practice: an incident-monitoring study. *Medical Journal of Australia* 1998; **169**: 73–6.

9 Blendon R J, Schoen C, Des Roches C, Osborn R and Zapert K. Common concerns amid diverse systems: health care experiences in five countries. *Health Affairs* 2003; **22**: 106–21.

10 Coulter A and Jenkinson C. European patients' views on the responsiveness of health systems and healthcare providers. *European Journal of Public Health* 2005. doi: 101093/eurpub/cko04.

11 General Medical Council. *Good Medical Practice*. London: GMC, 2001.

12 Royal College of General Practitioners and the General Practitioners Committee. *Good Medical Practice for General Practitioners*. London: RCGP, 2002.

13 WONCA Europe. *The European Definition of General Practice/Family Medicine*. London: WONCA Europe. 2002.

14 www.rcgp.org.uk/default.aspx?page=2561 [accessed September 2006].

Consultation models

History and histories

This chapter explores:

- early models of the consultation ● the concept of paternalism
- content and process; tasks and behaviours ● the contrast
between the biomedical and biopsychosocial models ● the patient-
centred approach ● the expert patient ● narrative-based medicine
- agendas ● issues relating to adopting the patient-centred approach.

It is mainly concerned with 'finding out', 'information gathering'
and 'sharing information'.

'It is a quite inexplicable frame of mind which prompts a person to consult a physician and then to conceal from the latter vital information; however, this is not at all infrequently the case.'

A F BYFIELD[1]

Consultations and the first doctor–patient interaction usually begin with the doctor 'taking' a medical history. In the traditional sense of history taking, the doctor seeks to find out why the patient has decided to consult, and explores the patient's symptoms in a logical and structured manner, gathering information in order to formulate a diagnosis.

○ **Consultation (from the Latin *consultare*)** *a conference between two or more people to consider a particular question.*

Of course, not all consultations involve a diagnosis-defining process. Increasingly primary care is concerned with the management of chronic conditions and screening for signs of early pathology. However, sharing information is a fundamental part of the majority of doctor–patient interactions and this chapter will concentrate on the process.

The medical history and early patient involvement

The medical history was and is the mainstay of any attempt at diagnosis and subsequent management, though, as will be discussed, terminology and process are changing as the study of the doctor–patient relationship and consultation skills evolve. As Roy Porter, an expert on the eighteenth- and nineteenth-century history of medicine, wrote: 'The reliance upon taking the history was a positive mark of the confidence felt by the expert clinician in his personal ability to assess a case solely from the patient's story and gross physical signs.'[2] Taking a full history could take well over half an hour[3] and events from considerable periods of time were often considered.[4] Indeed, such was the confidence in history taking, and the contemporary lack of expertise in examination, that consultations were often conducted by mail.[5] In 1752, the clinician John Rutherford wrote: 'We must learn the nature of a disease by an accurate and distinct account of it from the patients…to discover its causes and the part affected.'[6]

Physicians had to take into account the beliefs of their patients, many of whom had a wealth of concepts and remedies on which to draw. Moral, emotional and social factors were discussed in consultations as well as the physical details of the ailment. Medical knowledge was a part of the popular culture of the eighteenth century and patients expected to have a say in their treatment. In fact, the consultation of the time could be viewed as a negotiation about diagnosis and treatment between physician and patient.[2] However, records also show that the attitudes of doctors towards their patients ranged from subservience (usually to rich clients) to downright authoritarianism from the middle of the eighteenth century.[7]

Erosion of patient partnership and the rise of paternalism

○ **Paternalism** *the practice of treating people in a fatherly manner; providing for their needs without giving them rights or responsibilities.*

The partnership between doctor and patient started to erode in the mid-eighteenth century mainly because of the increasing use of the hospital as a site to treat the sick, particularly the sick lower classes. Thomas Percival (1740 – 1804) advocated reinforcing paternalism, especially as regards these poorer and charity patients, though he admitted that adopting an authoritarian stance towards paying patients might be more difficult.[8]

As doctors assumed control in hospitals with a subsequent increase in medical autonomy, the patient's narrative of illness became redundant. The nineteenth century saw a swing towards a more scientific basis for medicine with the establishment of scientific method and experiments,[9] which further undermined the doctor–patient partnership of the previous century. With the rise of scientific medicine the 'sick man' disappeared and the 'patient', a pathological body studded with lesions, made an appearance.[10] What went on in the consultation in these centuries is difficult to establish as the only evidence that remains is in the form of anecdotes relating doctor–patient encounters involving the upper classes. As science advanced, and doctors became more diagnostically and therapeutically powerful, the bedside manner was often forgotten, though bedside tools such as the stethoscope and ophthalmoscope meant that examining a patient became increasingly important. The physical examination became a bridge between the doctor's scientific knowledge and the patient's symptoms.[10]

Primary care, established in the middle of the nineteenth century in the United Kingdom, gave everyone the opportunity to see a doctor. The concept of the family doctor, with its overtones of a strong personal bond between doctor and patient, did not exist before the early part of the nineteenth century.[11] In contrast with the movement towards laboratory science in medicine and the increasing use of hospitals by physicians and patients, in the nineteenth century the general practitioner still continued to visit patients at home and to treat the 'whole person', with the patient retaining a degree of control over the consultation.[11]

The biomedical model: the disease-centred approach

○ **Biomedical** *relating to the activities and applications of science to clinical medicine.*

In modern times the history is still the cornerstone of the medical encounter though the process of 'taking a history' differs depending on the patient and the nature of the presenting complaint or symptoms that have prompted the patient to seek medical help. Taking a history in a formal and structured way, albeit in practice usually in a truncated form compared with that learnt at medical school, tends to make a consultation disease or doctor centred.[12] The components of the traditional medical history were defined in the first edition of *Clinical Methods* in 1897. This textbook, which became *Hutchison's Clinical Methods* and a favourite of British medical students, defined history taking as 'the interrogation of the patient'.[13] However, by 1929 the text advised letting the patient 'tell (the) story in his own words' and suggested that 'the use of leading questions is only occasionally allowable … it may also be necessary in dealing with patients who are stupid by nature or as the result of disease'.[14] Another late nineteenth-century text advised student or physician 'to listen attentively and as far as possible without interruption to the patient's own statement of his case' but suggested that the histories of the rich were reliable while those of the poor were not, and that to distrust or disregard the word of paying patients was professional suicide.[15] The case history, information to be gathered from the patient, was to include the elements listed in Box 2.1.

Box 2.1 ○ The traditional medical history

○ The presenting complaint.

○ History of the present illness.

○ Previous history of illness.

○ Menstrual history.

○ Treatment history.

○ Family history.

○ Social history.

○ Psychiatric history.

○ (Systems review.)

After an initial query from the doctor as to the nature of the problem and the patient's opening description of the symptoms, the doctor sets the agenda by asking questions in order to formulate a list of differential diagnoses or the most likely nature of the patient's problem. This method of information gathering is one-sided; an effect reinforced by the use of the word 'take' in the process of taking a history.

Medical students sometimes criticise patients for being 'poor historians'. This is usually a failure of the student to elicit a history by judicious use of communication skills.

However, it is true that patients' memories of their illnesses, past medical history and treatment are often patchy. When checked against a previous version of their story, dates may be different, severity of symptoms may change and sometimes events may be recalled that could not have happened. This lack of consistency may be important for diagnostic purposes and is likely to be more significant if the GP does not have access to full medical records including hospital letters and investigation results. I am often surprised at how little patients have been told about their conditions and drug treatments. Perhaps this is poor memory but it is also certainly due to poor sharing of information.

One US psychiatrist has suggested that histories may be more reliable if the patient is questioned in the same manner each time and by the doctor clarifying the exact meaning of common terms such as 'all the time', 'a lot' or 'several'.[16] To be fair to this doctor he does agree that in certain circumstances it is also important to obtain the patient's history in their own words.

In 1993 the sociologists Fisher and Todd suggested that the structure of the consultation reflects a mechanistic view focused on disease rather than health or prevention, arising from the germ theory of illness and the division of mind and body.[17] The biomedical model is limited because it does not take into account that health and illness are also shaped by personal and social as well as biological factors. This model leads to a disease-centred approach, where the main tasks of the doctor are to diagnose illness from a biological perspective and to treat it, hopefully effecting a cure. The drive to make a diagnosis is extremely strong. The biomedical model disconnects medicine from the social fabric of patients' lives.[18] The traditional history-taking format has also been criticised as being unproven in its effectiveness in improving medical conditions.[19]

Disease-centred consultations are also doctor centred and usually end with the doctor making a diagnosis and prescribing treatment. The patient is not involved in any management decisions and thus may not take the prescribed treatment correctly, if at all, or may seek another opinion. Doctor-centred consultations hinder compliance with treatment,[20] the term compliance in itself suggesting the power base of the transaction.

Doctor-centred behaviour also stems from the idea that there is a competence gap between the doctor and patient, i.e. the difference in the level of knowledge between doctor and patient, a gap that may be bridged by trust. In 1951 Parsons, a functionalist sociologist (i.e. someone who looks at how social institutions fill social needs) and professor at Harvard, wrote that illness is not strictly a pathophysiological process but is also a social phenomenon. When people become ill they adopt a sick role, behaviour that may be seen as a form of deviance. The doctor then acts as an agent of social control, either allowing or disallowing the patient's continuation of this role by the doctor's power of sick certification. In Parson's analysis, the doctor–patient relationship is a formal and distant one. The doctor is concerned only with the patient's health and less interested in matters that are not health-related.[21] The doctor expects the patient 'to obey' the doctor without question while the doctor gives the minimum amount of information to the patient.

Integrating content and process

Early work on involving patients in the consultation process, beyond merely asking a series of generally closed questions and then 'prescribing' what to do, included that of Balint, a psychoanalyst who worked with groups of general practitioners in the UK from the late 1950s. He focused on exploring the nature of the doctor–patient relationship and practical ways of reaching understanding of patients' illnesses.[22] Interestingly, the new edition of *Clinical Methods* in 1968 advised that patients were asked why they had come to the doctor or hospital at this particular time as the 'answer sometimes surprises'.[23] In 1974 the 16th edition reminded readers that 'History taking is still an art and a *special form of communication*' and that doctors should ask patients 'What made you decide to come and see me at this time?'[24] These types of questions mirror those that Helman, a medical anthropologist, suggested that patients seek answers to when they consult a doctor, for example 'Why is this happening to me and why now?'[25]

In the 1970s and 1980s doctors and sociologists began to dissect the nature of the consultation in more detail, looking at how doctors communicate with patients, in an attempt to define the tasks and behaviours of the consultation. Tasks are those areas that should be explored or discussed (content) while behaviours are how the doctor achieves them (process). Content and process have all too often been treated as separate entities. At an undergraduate medical education level, for instance, communication skills (process) have often been learned separately from history taking (content). Integration of the two in clinical skills teaching marries the task-orientated consultation with the patient-centred behavioural approach.[26]

Involving the patient: the biopsychosocial model and patient-centred care

Balint and his co-workers first used the term 'patient-centred medicine' in 1970, a reference to the client-centred therapy expounded by the psychologist Carl Rogers.[27] The term was contrasted with 'illness centred'. The British GPs Byrne and Long compared the patient-centred style with what they called the doctor-centred style of consulting.[28] In the latter the manner of consulting is based only on the doctor's knowledge and questioning of the patient in order to formulate a diagnosis, whereas the former incorporates the patient's experiences and health beliefs. In a patient-centred consultation the doctor and patient consider the patient's condition and diagnosis in partnership, and the management or treatment plan is negotiated between the doctor and patient.

The GPs Stott (now Professor of General Practice in Cardiff) and Davis emphasised the need within the consultation to combine clinical acumen with an insight into human behaviour.[29] They suggested that doctors need to develop skills in order to make a comprehensive assessment of the patient's problems: 'the integrated physical and psychosocial formulation is relevant to every speciality'. This formulation helps to widen the diagnostic process. They concluded that the tasks of the consultation encompass modification of health-seeking behaviour and opportunistic health promotion as well as the diagnosis and management of new and continuing problems.

In 1983 the psychologist Pendleton wrote that

> it would seem that satisfaction of the patient is more likely when the doctor discovers and deals with the patient's concerns and expectations; when the doctor's manner communicates warmth, interest and concern about the patients, when the doctor volunteers a lot of information and explains things to the patient in terms that are understood.[30]

The patient-centred approach to the consultation recognises that a patient's problem may be defined in terms of its physical, psychological and social components (the biopsychosocial model).[31,32] The cause of the problem, how the patient handles it and its course are determined by the patient's 'understanding of and emotional response to what is happening'.[33] Bensing, of the Department of Health Psychology at the Netherlands Institute of Primary Care, has defined psychosocial care as 'receptiveness for and treatment of the (aetiological and consequential) non-somatic aspects of the presented health problem'.[34] Thus, ultimately, a diagnosis may encompass more than a medical problem. The doctor needs to be aware of the nature and cause of the problem, and the reason for the patient seeking medical advice at the time, and should try to discover the patient's ideas, concerns and expectations.

The classic text of general practice literature, printed in 1984[33] and revised in 2003,[35] *The Consultation* by Pendleton and his colleagues, lists and describes the tasks of the consultation. With reference to 'finding out' it uses the terminology 'identifying the aetiology of the patient's problem' and includes considering 'at risk factors'.

The patient-centred clinical method

In Ontario, Canada, in 1986, a group of doctors working within the Department of Family Medicine described a model for the consultation that they also called 'the patient-centred clinical method'.[36] This method was defined and refined following an analysis of 1000 audiotaped consultations that had taken place in South Africa. They divided the consultations into 'effective' and 'less effective'. They demonstrated, reinforcing previous work, that one of the defining characteristics of the effective consultation was the doctor eliciting the patient's concerns and expectations. In less effective consultations the doctor failed to recognise or ignored the patient's agenda. The group also highlighted the need to find out why the patient was presenting at that time. Thus one part of the patient-centred model may be summarised as ICEE (Box 2.2).

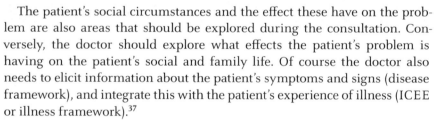

Box 2.2 ○ ICEE

The clinician explores:

○ the patient's *I*deas about what is wrong

○ the patient's feelings (*C*oncerns) about the illness(es)

○ the impact (*E*ffect) of the patient's problems on function/daily living

○ the patient's *E*xpectations about what should be done.

The patient's social circumstances and the effect these have on the problem are also areas that should be explored during the consultation. Conversely, the doctor should explore what effects the patient's problem is having on the patient's social and family life. Of course the doctor also needs to elicit information about the patient's symptoms and signs (disease framework), and integrate this with the patient's experience of illness (ICEE or illness framework).[37]

The patient-centred clinical method defines not only the information-gathering part of the consultation but also offers a framework for the latter stages of the consultation that will be dealt with in the next chapters. In terms of information gathering, defining the term 'patient centred' in a few words is difficult. The easiest approach is to say it involves putting the patient at the centre or focus of the consultation. But that is a tautology and unhelpful. The model embraces both abstract and concrete concepts, and requires a clinician to have not only certain skills but also the right attitude to patient care. Doctors need to exhibit a willingness to probe into areas of a patient's life that are not, on the face of it, relevant to the medical problem. This process has also been called 'building a history'.[38]

Another related concept that has been advocated mainly in the USA is relationship-centred care. This is defined as an approach to health care and healing that places relationship at the core of the therapeutic process.[39] All interactions are based upon a fundamental commitment to mutual respect, self-awareness, humility, openness and caring. Relationship building between health professional and patient is an important part of the process.[40] It is perhaps the logical next step after doctor centred and patient centred but the latter is still a more familiar term in the UK.

Curiosity and empathy are key attributes in the practice of a patient-centred approach. Empathy involves recognising when emotions may be present but not directly expressed, and the doctor acknowledging and exploring these unexpressed feelings so that the patient may feel understood.[41] Also important are the more prosaic skills of organisation and time management. Novice practitioners usually find a formalised structure helpful, with the tasks of the consultation clearly delineated. More experienced clinicians should be able to deviate from such a rigid path, acknowledging and working through both the patient's and their own agenda, while being mindful of the desired outcome of the consultation for both participants.

Ultimately the best way of measuring the patient centredness of a consultation is by asking patients themselves[42] (Box 2.3). The patient voice is a powerful but often neglected tool when evaluating consultations. It will be considered further in Chapters 7, 8 and 9.

Box 2.3 ○ What patients want from a consultation

○ Exploration of main reason for consultation.

○ Integrated understanding of patient's world (whole person, emotional needs, life issues).

○ Common ground as to nature of problem.

○ Mutual agreement on management.

○ Enhancement of health promotion and disease prevention.

○ Enhancement of doctor–patient relationship.

Evidence for the patient-centred approach

Learning and practising the patient-centred model should help doctors improve healthcare outcomes.[43] Effective information gathering using a patient-centred approach has been shown to improve such outcomes.[44] If the doctor asks many questions about the patient's understanding of the problem, explores concerns and expectations, and discusses the impact of the problem on daily life, there is better resolution of anxiety[45] and symptoms.[46] If the patient is able to express him or herself and feels that there has been a full discussion of the problem, physical limitation is reduced[47] and health status improves.[48]

The patient as expert

○ **Expert** *a person with special knowledge or skills who performs proficiently.*

In 1985 a group of social scientists at the Health Education Studies Unit in Cambridge published the results of their research study into medical consultations. The aim of the work was to study the extent to which ideas are shared between doctors and patients, in particular to look at what is said or done in consultations to help patients understand what is happening to them. The patient was defined as an expert about their illness. By asking about a patient's ideas about the illness or problem, the doctor would tap into this expertise and then share their own professional diagnosis of the problem in turn with the patient. Thus, while not mentioning patient centredness specifically, the approach is similar to that of the other workers already mentioned.

In conclusion Tuckett and his colleagues from Cambridge[49] argued that patients should be treated as experts. They defined that successful shared understanding had taken place if, following a consultation, a patient could remember the key points of what the doctor had said and be aware of points of conflict and difference with the doctor. Shared understanding leads onto shared decision making and the management phase of the consultation, which will be discussed in the next chapter.

Narrative-based medicine

○ **Narrative** *a message that tells the particulars of an act, occurrence or course of events.*

As described above, as medicine became more science based, the history-taking process moved away from the patient's narrative. There is now a movement to bring narrative back into the consultation so that the medical history once again becomes the patient's story. Greenhalgh and Hurwitz, academic GPs in London, suggest that 'the narrative context of illness provides a framework for approaching a patient's problem holistically, as well as revealing potential diagnostic and therapeutic options'.[50] Practitioners use ethnographic methodologies in listening to their patients in order to understand their stories. The main task of the narrative-based approach has been defined as helping patients to develop new stories, 'a shared new narrative'.[51] It can be argued that the narrative-based medicine movement is another way of suggesting that patients should be asked to describe their problems in their own words, and within their own context, and that the doctor's communication skills should facilitate this process.

How does this then differ from the patient-centred approach? We need to be careful of establishing a new jargon and new terms, many of which have overlapping meanings but which may also become confusing for the practising doctor. Given that we are thinking about communication, it is paradoxical that our own terminology may cloud understanding.

The presenting complaint and the patient's agenda

○ **Agenda** *an organised plan for matters to be attended to; a list of matters to be taken up (as at a meeting).*

One practitioner of narrative-based primary care believes that patient-centred care has itself become too prescriptive and that the exploration of the patient's ideas, concerns and expectations has become a part of the doctor's agenda, which may in fact ignore the patient's agenda. Moreover he criticises the patient-centred approach for assuming that the patient's agenda is fixed and predetermined, while a story-centred approach starts from the premise that a patient is seeking an agenda.[51]

However, the more widely accepted view at present is that most patients come to the consultation with a particular agenda, which encompasses ICEE, and that this needs to be explored. Nevertheless, the doctor must remember that this exploration serves a purpose and is not just an item in the consultation to be ticked off as done. When a patient decides to consult a general practitioner they usually have a reason for making the appointment or going to the surgery. This may be a traditional 'presenting complaint' in that the patient has developed a symptom or disability that needs to be diagnosed and/or managed. Often the patient is seeking something else, for example a repeat prescription for an ongoing condition, a medical certificate or advice. This reason is the patient's agenda at that moment. However, by the time the patient arrives at the consultation other issues may have arisen that they want to discuss. Some patients wait for several days before they can see a doctor of their choice in their practice. The original problem may have resolved but they still decide to consult. Thus the patient's agenda is flexible. A GP may open a consultation with the words 'What seems to be the problem?' but these are often inappropriate unless there is a definite presenting complaint. A more useful and profitable greeting may be 'What may I do for you today?' Practitioners will find their own style.

Neighbour, in his influential book *The Inner Consultation*, addresses the subject of the patient's opening remarks, stating that the first thing a patient says is the only part of the consultation over which they have much control[52] (though the process of shared decision making, which is discussed in Chapter 3, does give more control to patients). Patients rehearse what they plan to say and begin with what Neighbour calls the opening gambit, though sometimes this is preceded by a more spontaneous remark, the curtain raiser.[52] The gambit is the overt agenda. An uninterrupted patient will usually conclude the opening monologue within 30 seconds but physicians often interject before the end; this only results in shortening the monologue by about 10 seconds.[53]

There is also the 'hidden agenda'. This covert agenda is often not the 'presenting complaint' or stated reason for the consultation as mentioned first by the patient.[54] If the doctor decides to focus on the initial concern or problem, interrupting the patient too early, the patient's late-arising concerns are rarely completely described. This means that the doctor misses an opportunity to gather potentially important information.[55] Patients may then introduce an unmet need via the 'doorknob' comment, i.e. something mentioned as the patient is about to leave the room.[56] This may be the patient's last attempt to raise an issue and may be disregarded by a time-pressurised physician.

Vocational training programmes and even undergraduate medical school communication skills teaching place a great emphasis on the 'hidden agenda'. While this is laudable and necessary, there is a danger that inexperienced doctors will seek a hidden agenda in most consultations, particularly when being assessed. Patients are asked repeatedly 'Is there anything else I can do for you?' We need to accept that sometimes the 'presenting complaint' or stated reason for the consultation is all that the patient wishes to discuss on this occasion and not almost bully the patient into divulging other information that is irrelevant or inappropriate at this point. Moreover the desire to 'do something else' for the patient may hinder the doctor and patient working through the issues that the patient has already brought up.

Issues relating to patient-centred care

Despite the criticisms of the patient-centred approach, it is this process that informs much of the learning and teaching on the consultation today. However, there are potential problems for practitioners in developing this approach. Doctors report greater satisfaction with consultations if they only have to deal with simple patient agendas.[57] Lack of confidence makes them reluctant to tackle complex agendas.[58] Doctors may be overwhelmed by the scope and nature of their patients' problems even if they are able and willing to explore ideas, concerns and expectations fully. They may feel powerless in the face of certain patient expectations and previously unmet needs (see Chapter 7 for a further discussion of this issue). Moreover pressures on time and short consultation lengths, such as the UK average of 9.36 minutes,[59] can increase the reluctance of general practitioners to engage with patients in this way. Social and emotional issues are often neglected in consultations for all these reasons.[60] However, given that patient-centred interviews appear to increase patient satisfaction and outcomes,[61] as well as resulting in fewer investigations and referrals,[42] such consultations may be more cost-effective in the long term.

Doctors do not stick to one method of consulting and move between the patient centred and the doctor centred for many reasons as well as time management. A tired or burnt-out GP is less likely to engage with patients on an emotional level. Doctors with personal problems of their own may find it difficult, paradoxically, to empathise with a patient with family, work or social problems. A difficult consultation with a patient during a previous encounter will affect the performance of the doctor when interacting with that same patient on a subsequent occasion. Similarly a doctor's own values and beliefs will affect the way a consultation is conducted.[33] It is important that GPs recognise these influences and try not to let them affect patient care adversely.

Modern GPs are asked to consider discussing health promotion and disease prevention, including screening, during appropriate consultations. These tasks often bring in increased remuneration as well as contributing in part to the public health. Such issues may not be part of a patient's expectations and thus it needs to be asked if they can be considered as part of a patient-centred process. Of course some patients wish to engage with the doctor on these issues and this should be explored. However, the doctor's and the public health agenda may not be something that the patient wishes to consider on a particular occasion. Therefore we think that the doctor should consequently give the patient space to decline such interventions without prejudice. Notes are often written that state that a patient refused treatment, immunisation, screening, etc. The word 'refuses/refused' has overtones of the doctor-centred worldview and the word 'declines/declined' is more appropriate.

Patients may also be unused to interacting with doctors in a patient-centred way. Many worry about wasting the doctor's time with problems they perceive as non-medical.[34] Even if asked to share ideas and concerns, patients may find it difficult to express their feelings, especially if they are not used to articulating their thoughts. Some patients with a relatively straightforward agenda may feel uncomfortable if asked about issues they regard as unrelated to that agenda. Obviously patient and doctor factors interact when considering the success or otherwise of a consultation. Skilled doctors are more able to put patients at their ease and facilitate two-way communication, explaining why they are asking certain questions and probing into certain areas. On balance, patients, particularly those with psychosocial problems, do want a patient-centred approach with a doctor who communicates well.[62]

However, on occasion some patients will want a quick consultation with a doctor that addresses their needs promptly. Defining and addressing these needs are patient centred but in a truncated way. In a group practice patients will often choose a particular doctor to provide the type of consultation they want. These are factors that need to be considered when advocating adoption of this model and when defining training needs for doctors (Table 2.1). Doctors should be cautious of slavishly following guidelines without reflecting on the process. *There is a danger that exploring ICEE may become rote behaviour without any engagement with the process, and thus the exploration becomes another task on a checklist.*

Ideas, concerns and expectations ○ *reflections*

I remember one of my rare visits to my GP. I saw a doctor I'd never met as a patient, though I knew his name as one of the GP undergraduate teachers. He asked me what I made of my persistent cough, while examining me. I said 'I suppose it is just a hangover from a cold and cough I had some weeks ago. It's just that it's been going on so long. ...' 'And do you have any concerns about it?' 'Well,' I laughed, feeling daft yet relieved, 'in the night I worry it's cancer. ...' He finished checking details. He told me, 'Yes, it is a leftover from the cold, there is no infection and the bronchus can remain irritated after a virus. It's not likely to be cancer as you have not lost weight. So you'll have to carry on, I'm afraid. It should wear off soon, may take a while, come back if it doesn't. Anything else you expected from seeing me today?'

He did all he needed to do and so did I, in about four minutes. I'd been ICEd. It works. It seems simple but we all struggle with being direct like this.

Table 2.1 ○ **Factors hindering adoption of patient-centred approach**

Doctor factors	Organisational factors
Lack of training	Lack of time
Lack of empathy	Payment structure
Emphasis on tasks rather than process	Lack of support
Reluctance to explore patient concerns	Lack of resources to meet patient needs
Powerless in face of patient expectations	Pressure from other doctors to see more patients
Burnout	Poor conditions
Inability to cope with uncertainty	
Inability to cope with change	
Following guidelines without reflection	

Patient factors	Doctor and patient factors
Worry about wasting doctor's time	Language barriers
Concern about appropriateness of consultation	Cultural differences
Worry about being able to express their problem	
Embarrassment about the situation	
Being in an artificial environment	
Sense of failure due to having to consult about the problem	

Patient-centred consultations ○ *reflections*

Looking back on my experiences as a GP (trainee) registrar and then vocation-ally trained GP for 20 years I realise that in the early years I was a particularly doctor-centred practitioner. Diagnosis and disease management were the focus of the doctor–patient interaction. I was a shy medical student and hid behind the structure of the biomedical history-taking model. This seemed to serve me well as a house officer and subsequent hospital-based junior doctor. Moving out into general practice – the career I had chosen from the moment I decided to be a doctor – was an unnerving experience. Where were the illnesses I knew? Some patients just seemed to want a chat. My trainer and his partners helped me understand some of the undercurrents of consultation patterns. Videotaping was in its infancy. We trainees squirmed at our incompetence on screen. We mapped our consultations, but somehow I missed the point. I couldn't deal with uncertainty and I found it hard to elicit any personal stories from 'my' patients until I had known them a while. And remember, by the time I became MRCGP, I was consulting at six-minute intervals.

When I wasn't stressed, when I wasn't on-call and anxious about being called out of surgery, and when I stopped thinking about being an efficient doctor, I relaxed into enjoying discovering what the patients were really saying. Patients began to tell me their concerns without my asking, but once I realised how use-ful this was, I did begin to ask.

I rediscovered the consultation skills literature when I became a trainer. I found it liberating to ask patients what they wanted from a consultation – get-ting straight to the point but in a roundabout way. The frustration then was only having seven minutes, later increased to 10. I now enjoy standard 15-minute consultations in Australia. The pressure is off and there is a chance to talk with patients. I feel able to hear their stories; perhaps this is a narrative-based approach. We GP academics may praise the patient-centred approach but I real-ise the problems of time and other pressures. Part of the issue is understanding fully what being patient centred is: not feeling guilty if consultations aren't perfect; being aware that the consultation is the patients' time and as doctors we are facilitators of how they spend that time.

Sometimes I do wonder what became of the simple approach: making a diag-nosis. But that process relates to my hospital posts when a patient was given a diagnosis and treated, or referred on to someone else who might know what was wrong. In the community diagnoses are often more difficult; cause and effect are entwined with an individual's circumstances. There are of course consultations that are straightforward. This is a cold caused by a virus. The patient wants advice. I don't think I am missing anything in the story. I remem-ber being told about the GP registrar who tried to explore the sexual history of every patient with a sore throat. Patients chose to see a different doctor the next time they had a cold. The registrar was being thorough but not sensitive to the needs of the patient. Some stories are short and simple; some are long and com-plicated. Experience and skills help us distinguish between the types, though we often still get it wrong.

○ **Summary**

- The patient-centred approach to consultations is now widely adopted as the method of information gathering/sharing of choice.

- However, it should not be followed slavishly as a rule but rather as a guideline to doctor–patient interactions.

- The agendas and consulting styles of both doctors and patients vary from one consultation to another.

- Not all patients on every encounter wish to discuss concerns or personal problems.

- The skill of the doctor is in eliciting a patient's needs on each particular occasion and checking that this is what the patient expects.

REFERENCES

1 Byfield A F. Case history taking. In: Tice F (ed). *Practice of Medicine. Volume 1.* Maryland: W F Prior, 1924. Chapter 12.

2 Porter R. The rise of physical examination. In: Bynum WF and Porter R (eds). *Medicine and the Five Senses.* Cambridge: Cambridge University Press, 1993, pp. 179–97.

3 Lane J. The doctor scolds me: the diaries and correspondence of patients in eighteenth century England. In: Porter R (ed.) *Patients and Practitioners.* Cambridge: Cambridge University Press, 1985, pp. 207–47.

4 Fissell M E. *Patients, Power and the Poor in Eighteenth-Century Bristol.* Cambridge: Cambridge University Press, 1991.

5 Porter D and Porter R. *Patient's Progress: Doctors and Doctoring in Eighteenth Century England.* Stanford: Stanford University Press, 1989.

6 Rutherford J. *Clinical Lectures.* MS 4217. London: Wellcome Institute, 1752.

7 Loudon I. *Medical Care and the General Practitioner 1750–1850.* Oxford: Clarendon Press, 1986.

8 Percival T. *A Handbook of Medical Ethics.* London: Russell & Johnson, 1803.

9 Bernard C. *An Introduction to the Study of Experimental Medicine.* New York: Dover Publications, 1957 [first published in 1865].

10 Porter R. *The Greatest Benefit to Mankind. A Medical History of Humanity from Antiquity to the Present.* London: Harper Collins, 1997.

11 Loudon I. The concept of the family doctor. *Bulletin of the History of Medicine* 1984; **58**: 347–62.

12 Stevens J. Brief encounter. Factors and fallacies in learning and teaching the science of consultation for the future general practitioner. *Journal of the Royal College of General Practitioners* 1974; **24**: 5–22.

13 Hutchison R and Rainey H. *Clinical Methods*. London: Cassell & Co, 1897.

14 Hutchison R and Hunter D. *Clinical Methods*. Ninth edition. London: Cassell & Co, 1929.

15 Bury J. *Clinical Medicine*. London: Charles Griffith, 1894.

16 Barsky A J. Forgetting, fabricating and telescoping. The instability of the medical history. *Archives of Internal Medicine* 2002; **162**: 981–4.

17 Fisher S and Todd A D. Introduction: communication and social context – toward broader definitions. In: Todd A D and Fisher S (eds). *The Social Organization of Doctor–Patient Communication*. New Jersey: Ablex Publishing Corporation, 1993, pp. 1–16.

18 Mishler E G. Viewpoint: critical perspectives on the biomedical model. In: Mishler E G, Amarasingham L R, Hauser S T, Liem R, Osherson S D and Waxler N (eds). *Social Contexts of Health, Illness and Patient Care*. Cambridge: Cambridge University Press, 1981.

19 Waitzkin H. *The Politics of Medical Encounters*. New Haven: Yale University Press, 1991.

20 Royal Pharmaceutical Society of Great Britain. *From Compliance to Concordance. Achieving Shared Goals in Medicine Taking*. London: R P S G B, 1997.

21 Parsons T. *The Social System*. London: Routledge & Kegan Paul, 1951.

22 Balint M. *The Doctor, His Patient and the Illness*. London: Tavistock Publications, 1957.

23 Hunter D and Bomford R R. *Hutchison's Clinical Methods*. Fifteenth edition. London: Cassell & Co, 1968.

24 Bomford R R, Mason S and Swash M. *Hutchison's Clinical Methods*. Sixteenth edition. London: Baillière Tindall, 1974.

25 Helman C G. Diseases versus illness in general practice. *Journal of the Royal College of General Practitioners* 1981; **31**: 548–52.

26 Kurtz S, Silverman J, Benson J and Draper J. Marrying content and process in clinical method teaching: enhancing the Calgary–Cambridge guides. *Academic Medicine* 2003; **78**: 802–9.

27 Rogers C R. *Client-Centred Therapy: Its Current Practice, Implications and Theory*. Boston: Houghton Mifflin, 1951.

28 Byrne P S and Long B E L. *Doctors Talking to Patients*. London: H M S O, 1967.

29 Stott N C and Davis R H. The exceptional potential in each primary care consultation. *Journal of the Royal College of General Practitioners* 1979; **29**: 201–5.

30 Pendleton D. Doctor–patient communication: a review. In: Pendleton D and Hasler J (eds) *Doctor–Patient Communication*. London: Academic Press, 1983.

31 Engel G L. A unified concept of health and disease. *Perspectives in Biology and Medicine* 1960; **3**: 459–85.

32 Engel G L. The clinical application of the biopsychosocial model. *American Journal of Psychiatry* 1980; **137**: 535–43.

33 Pendleton D, Schofield T, Tate P and Havelock P. *The Consultation: An Approach to Learning and Teaching.* Oxford: Oxford University Press, 1984.

34 Bensing J. Doctor–patient communication and the quality of care. *Social Science and Medicine* 1991; **32**: 1301–10.

35 Pendleton D, Schofield T, Tate P and Havelock P. *The New Consultation. Developing Doctor–Patient Communication.* Oxford: Oxford University Press, 2003.

36 Levenstein J H, McCracken E C, McWhinney I R, *et al.* The patient-centred clinical method. 1. A model for the doctor–patient interaction in family medicine. *Family Practice* 1986; **3**: 24–30.

37 Stewart M and Roter D. *Communicating with Medical Patients.* Newbury: Sage Publications, 1989.

38 Haidet P and Paterniti D A. 'Building' a history rather than 'taking' one: a perspective on information sharing during the medical interview. *Archives of Internal Medicine* 2003; **163**: 1134–40.

39 Brody H. Relationship-centered care: beyond the finishing school. *Journal of the American Board of Family Practice* 1995; **8**: 416–18.

40 Malloch K, Sluyter D and Moore N. Relationship-centered care: achieving true value in healthcare. *Journal of Nursing Administration* 2000; **30**: 379–85.

41 Suchman A L, Markakis K, Beckman H B and Frankel R. A model of empathic communication in the medical interview. *Journal of the American Medical Association* 1997; **277**: 678–82.

42 Stewart M. Towards a global definition of patient centred care. *BMJ* 2001; **322**: 444–5.

43 Stewart M, Brown J B, Donner A, *et al.* The impact of patient-centred care on outcomes. *Journal of Family Practice* 2002; **49**: 796–804.

44 Stewart M. Effective physician–patient communication and health outcomes: a review. *Canadian Medical Association Journal* 1995; **152**: 1423–33.

45 Evans B J, Kiellerup F D, Stanley R O, *et al.* A communication skills programme for increasing patients' satisfaction with general practice consultations. *British Journal of Medical Psychology* 1987; **60**: 373–8.

46 Haezen-Klemens I and Lapinska E. Doctor–patient interaction, patients' health behaviour and effects of treatment. *Social Science and Medicine* 1984; **19**: 9–18.

47 Greenfield S, Kaplan S and Ware J E. Expanding patient involvement in care – effects on patient outcomes. *Annals of Internal Medicine* 1985; **102**: 520–8.

48 Kaplan S H, Greenfield S and Ware J E. Assessing the effects of physician–patient interactions on the outcomes of chronic disease. *Medical Care* 1989; **275**: 5110–27.

49 Tuckett D, Boulton M, Olson C and Williams A. *Meetings with Experts. An Approach to Sharing Ideas in Medical Consultations.* London: Tavistock Publications, 1985.

50 Greenhalgh T and Hurwitz B. Why study narrative? In: Greenhalgh T and Hurwitz B (eds). *Narrative Based Medicine*. London: BMJ Books, 1998, pp. 3–29.

51 Launer J. *Narrative-Based Primary Care. A Practical Guide*. Abingdon: Radcliffe Medical Press, 2002.

52 Neighbour R. *The Inner Consultation*. Lancaster: MTP Press, 1987.

53 Rabinowitz I, Luzzatti R, Tamir A and Reis S. Length of patient's monologue, rate of completion and relation to other components of the clinical encounter: observational intervention study in primary care. *BMJ* 2004; **328**: 501–2.

54 McKinley R K and Middleton J F. What do patients want from doctors? Content analysis of written patient agendas for the consultation. *BJGP* 1999; **49**: 796–800.

55 Marvel M K, Epstein R M, Flowers K and Beckman HB. Soliciting the patient's agenda: have we improved? *Journal of the American Medical Association* 1999; **281**: 283–7.

56 Weston W W, Brown J B and McWilliam C L. Being realistic. In: Brown J B, Stewart M and Weston W W (eds). *Challenges and Solutions in Patient-Centered Care. A Case Book*. Oxford: Radcliffe Medical Press, 2002, pp. 183–8.

57 Winefield H R, Murrell T G C, Clifford J V, *et al*. The usefulness of distinguishing different types of general practice consultation, or are needed skills always the same? *Family Practice* 1995; **12**: 402–7.

58 Barry C A, Bradley C P, Britten N, *et al*. Patients' unvoiced agendas in general practice consultations: qualitative study. *BMJ* 2000; **320**: 1246–50.

59 Royal College of General Practitioners. *RCGP Information Sheet No 3: Consultation Length and Waiting Times*. London: RCGP, 2001.

60 Campion P D, Butler N M and Cox A D. Principle agendas of doctors and patients in general practice consultations. *Family Practice* 1992; **9**: 181–90.

61 Stewart M. What is a successful doctor–patient interview? A study of interactions and outcomes. *Social Science and Medicine* 1984; **19**: 167–75.

62 Little P, Everitt H, Williamson I, *et al*. Preferences of patients for patient centred approach to consultation in primary care: observational study. *BMJ* 2001; **322**: 468–74.

Shared decision making and patient partnership

Involving patients in management

This chapter explores:

- the process of sharing information with patients
- the concept of the expert patient ● issues relating to patient autonomy
- informed consent ● informed shared decision making
- patient partnership ● compliance and concordance.

The focus is on how to share information with patients, how to involve patients in management decisions and why these processes are important.

'Perform calmly and adroitly, concealing more things from the patient while you are attending to him … sometimes reprove sharply and emphatically, and sometimes comfort with solicitude and attention, revealing nothing of the patient's future or present condition.'

HIPPOCRATES[1]

Hippocrates wrote the above in the 5th century BCE, a clear instruction to physicians of the importance of paternalism as applied to sharing information. In Chapter 2 we discussed the concept of paternalism and mentioned the importance of doctor and patient sharing information. A simple model of the consultation involves the doctor gathering information from the patient in order to formulate a diagnosis, and then the doctor formulating a management plan in order to treat or hopefully cure the patient's problem(s) and/or presenting complaints.

Sharing information and ideas

As discussed previously, the patient-centred approach may be used to gather information, but having elicited the patients' concerns and ideas, doctors are still in the position of deciding how much information to give patients about their condition and possible management. The quantity and quality of this information affects how patients make decisions relating to their own health care and may limit their choice of treatment depending on the number of options they are given. In earlier texts for the teaching of communication skills, British physician Fletcher[2] and GPs Walton and colleagues[3] gave similar recommendations as to what doctors should routinely tell patients in consultations (Box 3.1). The patient appears to be a passive participant in the process.

Box 3.1 ○ **Suggested information to give to patients**
○ The possible diagnosis.
○ Necessary investigations and what they involve.
○ What the investigations might show.
○ The treatment.
○ The likely outcome of treatment.

Eliot Freidson, a US sociologist and notable critic of the medical profession, suggested in 1970 that doctors purposefully withhold information from patients in order to maintain their professional dominance and power.[4] This stems from their 'splendid isolation' from society at large and leads to the exertion of an unreasonable level of social control.[5] While many may disagree with this motive and feel that times have changed, doctors have been shown frequently to be poor at giving information, whether this is information about the illness[6] or information following a procedure. It is not only an inability to communicate to patients in the appropriate language and detail that causes problems, but also doctors' value judgements about what patients should be told. Doctors underestimate the amount of information patients wish to receive about the nature and cause of their problem, the likely course of the illness and its prognosis.[7] Patients expect to receive more detailed information about adverse events during operations than doctors are happy to deliver.[8] This may be partly due to the fact that doctors want to spare patients from information that the patients might find upsetting; and partly to doctors not wanting to have to deal with their own emotions when patients are upset (see Chapter 7 for more on this). But doctors display biases when deciding on a patient's best interests in this way, biases arising from a patient's gender, race and socio-economic status.[9]

Doctors also fail to communicate because of pressures on time and the difficulty of the task. They are reluctant to risk losing a patient's trust and possibly being sued, yet poor communication itself has been shown to increase the likelihood of malpractice suits.[10] In 1989 Roter, a social scientist now at Johns Hopkins University, suggested that the skill of a doctor in information giving is paramount for patient compliance and recall. 'Information-giving may be viewed as enhancing patient power and increasing the patient's ability to participate actively in the therapeutic process.'[11]

Medical students soon learn their new language of medical practice. The rate of their incorporating medical jargon into conversation is interesting to observe. Jargon is an important barrier to patient understanding. We are all guilty of misusing the English language and obscuring our meanings with abbreviations and technical terms, though thankfully with not so many Latin words as in the past. However, even everyday words may confuse patients if used in an unusual context or without adequate explanation.[12] The same word may have a very different connotation when spoken by a doctor as compared with a layperson. Think of *shock, stool* and *stomach*.

The patient-centred approach for information sharing

Moira Stewart and her co-workers in Western Ontario have defined six interactive components for the patient-centred clinical method (Box 3.2).[13] Components 1 and 2 are related broadly to information gathering. Component 3 is concerned with information sharing to reach shared or mutual understanding, and thus for doctor and patient ultimately to agree on a management plan.

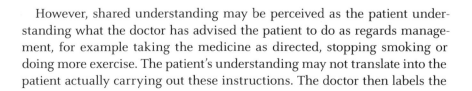

Box 3.2 ○ The patient-centred clinical method[13]

① Exploring both the disease and the illness experience (including ICEE).

② Understanding the whole person.

③ Finding common ground regarding management.

④ Incorporating prevention and health promotion.

⑤ Enhancing the doctor–patient relationship.

⑥ Being realistic.

However, shared understanding may be perceived as the patient understanding what the doctor has advised the patient to do as regards management, for example taking the medicine as directed, stopping smoking or doing more exercise. The patient's understanding may not translate into the patient actually carrying out these instructions. The doctor then labels the patient as non-compliant and wonders at the behaviour of these people who seek advice and do not follow it. Thus a patient-centred approach may revert to a doctor-centred approach in the latter stages of a consultation.

Models of the doctor–patient relationship: affecting management

The need to address the issue of poor compliance has led to research on why patients do not always do as their doctor advises and on ways in which to improve compliance. According to the patient-centred model, the doctor and patient should make management decisions in partnership,[14] thus aiding compliance with treatment and improving the outcome for the patient.[15] Of course, we should expect such management decisions to be affected by the patient's concerns and expectations as elicited during the history taking.

This partnership between doctor and patient is only one model of the doctor–patient relationship. There are a number of descriptions of the relationship based on the locus of control within it. In 1956 Szasz and Hollender, a psychiatrist and paediatrician respectively, provided an early discussion of three theoretical models of doctor–patient relationship. They suggested that which one of these is uppermost at any particular time depends on the nature of the patient's problem and the setting of the consultation.[16] The models are graded from the doctor being active while the patient is passive (*activity–passivity*) via the patient having limited power while being expected to co-operate with the doctor's advice (*guidance–co-operation*) to there being a state of *mutual participation*. This last model is the most difficult to sustain. Doctor and patient must be aware of the other's needs, wishes and individuality.

Over 30 years later the social scientists Roter and Hall wrote about the spectrum of high and low control.[17] There are four possible combinations of such control between physician and patient. High physician control combined with low patient control leads to a consultation in which the doctor dominates and makes decisions. The patient should co-operate with medical advice and do what they are told. This traditional form is paternalistic and may be described as patients drawing comfort and support from the doctor as a 'parent figure'.

Informed or independent choice and patient autonomy

○ **Autonomy** *'A form of personal liberty of action where the individual determines his or her own course of action in accordance with a plan chosen by him or herself.'*[18]

At the other end of the spectrum from paternalism, the physician adopts a completely neutral stance and gives the patient a range of options without expressing any preference, the 'informed model'[19] (independent choice). Here there is low physician control combined with high patient control. This model has been seen as a move towards increased patient autonomy. The rationale is that patients should be free to decide on an option without being contaminated by the doctor's experience or other social forces. One could say that this is the ultimately patient-centred model. Patients are not biased by the doctor's personal recommendation.[20] After the patient has decided, it is up to the doctor to implement that choice.

However, the informed model has been criticised as sacrificing competence for consumerism because of the fact that physicians withhold their own experience and recommendations to avoid overly influencing patients.[21] 'Too often autonomous patients and families are asked to make critical medical decisions on the basis of neutrally presented statistics, as free as possible from the contaminating influences of physicians.'[21] In contrast Quill, of the Department of Medicine at the University of Rochester in New York, and Brody, of the Department of Family Practice at Michigan University, have suggested that enhancing patient autonomy requires that doctors engage in open dialogue with patients, fully informing them of the options for treatment, with all their attendant advantages and disadvantages. However, doctors should also offer recommendations that consider both the doctors' and the patients' sets of values, health beliefs and experiences.[21] Not surprisingly they call this the enhanced autonomy model. This model is 'relationship centred' (a concept mentioned briefly in Chapter 2) lying as it does between doctor centred and patient centred. Both doctor and patient, and sometimes family members or carers, are included in the decision-making process.[22] Doctors should have genuine concern about their patients' best interests. They should support and guide patients' decision making without surrendering the medical power on which patients depend.[21]

Whether doctors should keep their medical power intact is an interesting question. Power may be thought of in three dimensions: in the first dimension A forces B to do something; in the second A controls the agenda in any interaction with B; in the third A controls the world as B sees it. The third dimensional view of power is relevant to the decision-making process.[23]

B (the patient) will make a decision based on the information received from A (the doctor). Thus B's actions are shaped by the medical knowledge supplied by A. B may have a free choice of options, but only of those options that A has decided to supply. A, in fact, still holds the balance of power within the doctor–patient relationship. Canter, a consultant surgeon in an editorial in the *British Medical Journal*, suggests that doctors usually supply information based firmly within a conventional biomedical framework. Choices involving alternative or complementary treatments are often ignored. He suggests that 'when the exercise of clinical power shifts from crude, but easily recognisable, coercive or first dimensional power to the more subtle and harder to recognise third dimensional power, the reality is that nothing may have changed'.[24]

The power still remains within the consultation with the doctor, who decides how much and what sort of information to share. In some situations this decision is informed by law, under the doctrine of informed consent.

Informed consent

Before considering decision making in the consultation further, it is important to look at the development of the allied concept of informed consent. This concept has evolved over the centuries from ancient times, when physicians expected absolute obedience from their patients, to a more liberal view of patients needing certain information about risk in order to consent to operations or invasive procedures. Except in emergencies, doctors who acted without patients' consent were at first accused of battery or intentional harm and later of negligence. Such consent has been a legal concept since 1767 in the UK, though at that time a doctor only had to inform a patient of the nature of a medical procedure. If the patient then submitted voluntarily to that procedure consent was implied. The term 'informed consent' itself was first used in a Californian court in 1957.

Informed consent is really about risk communication (further discussed in Chapter 4). However, when considering sharing information it is helpful for a doctor to consider the 'reasonable person standard'. This concept, established in the USA in 1972, states that a doctor's decision about whether a patient should have been informed of a risk is based on whether a reasonable person in that patient's position would want to be informed.[25] How a general practitioner may make such a judgement is a key question in the shared decision-making process.

An eloquent account of the tension between minimal sharing of information and absolute disclosure of all possible adverse effects by doctors is given in Jay Katz's book *The Silent World of Doctor and Patient*, published in 1984.[26] Katz is a physician and law professor at Yale University. His thesis is that doctors wish to preserve the mystique of their profession and believe that lay incompetence in relation to medical matters means that only a limited amount of explanation is needed for patient agreement to treatment. The rise of scientific method and the regulation and rationalisation of medical education in the 19th century led to an expansion in knowledge and concomitant professionalisation of medical practice. While this expansion in medical knowledge has meant improvements in life expectancy and reduced morbidity, Katz feels that 'the affirmation of physician's commitment to patients' physical needs ... [has] failed to address physicians' lack of commitment to patients' decision making needs'.[26]

However, these requirements are not so clear within everyday general practice and in relation to prescribing or other management decisions. How many side effects do GPs list for patients prior to prescribing? The big question remains: how much information do GPs give to patients? Furthermore, are we comfortable with the idea of patient autonomy and the possibility that doctors' patients will decline to follow management plans?

Informed shared decision making

In the UK we talk about the shared model to convey these concepts. This model, which incorporates the notions of the patient as partner and management by negotiation, is now in the ascendancy. It has become part of UK national policy as defined by the National Health Service Executive.[27] However, it should be noted that there is often difficulty in distinguishing between shared decision making and informed choice, and that separating the two models may not be actually justified in practice.[28] The term informed shared decision making (ISDM) has been used to combine the two models.[29]

Moreover, as highlighted above, sharing decisions is not simply sharing information. The skills needed for sharing decision making, usually in the 'second half of the consultation', have often been neglected at the expense of the information-gathering and information-sharing stages.[30] Yet two decades ago Katz gave a succinct account of the process in a reply to a colleague. This colleague could discuss options with other doctors but felt that patients would not be able to comprehend or tolerate the choices and their attendant uncertainties. Katz wrote of how he would interact with a patient when discussing treatment options for breast cancer:

I would have first clearly acknowledged our ignorance about which treatment is best. I would then have laid out all treatment modalities in considerable detail and discussed them with the patient. Eventually I would have made a recommendation but only after I had first elicited her preference *and* the reasons for her choice. Holding back for a while on giving her my recommendation would have served two purposes: one, to prevent her being pressured by my professional authority to accept my recommendation; and two, to provide an additional opportunity to explore … why she had chosen that particular treatment. We would then have been better situated to clarify whether her decision was affected by a lack of understanding of what I had said or whether I had insufficiently appreciated her wishes, needs and expectations.[26]

Thirteen years later Cathy Charles – a social scientist and health economist of McMaster University in Canada – and colleagues have defined a model of shared decision making that has four main characteristics (Box 3.3). For such shared decision making to be carried out in practice the commitment of both doctor and patient to engage in the process is crucial, although the extent of involvement may vary.

Box 3.3 ○ Characteristics of shared decision making[31]

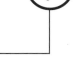

① Both the patient and the doctor are involved.

② Both parties share information.

③ Both parties take steps to build a consensus about the preferred treatment.

④ Doctor and patient reach an agreement on the treatment to implement.

The Informed Shared Decision Making Project of the University of British Columbia in Vancouver, led by Angela Towle, has suggested a series of steps that should occur in consultations that would enable doctors and patients to share in the decision-making process (Box 3.4). A list of ISDM competencies for doctors is derived from these steps (Box 3.5).[32]

A fundamental step in the ISDM process is the decision by the doctor as to which management options should be described. The ideas of the doctor as to the correct course of action will obviously colour their choice of which options to present to the patient. Doctors may choose the amount and type of information they give in order to influence patients' choices.[33] The options may be limited by the doctor's lack of knowledge in a particular field, or by previous experience of a treatment causing an adverse reaction in a patient.

Box 3.4 ○ Steps to ensure doctor and patient share in decision making[32]

① Establish a context in which patients' views about treatment options are valued and necessary.

② Elicit patients' preferences so that appropriate treatment options are discussed.

③ Transfer technical information to the patient on the treatment options, risks and probable benefits in an unbiased, clear and simple way.

④ Physician participation includes helping the patient conceptualise the weighing process of risks versus benefits and ensuring that their preferences are based on fact and not misconception.

⑤ Shared decision making involves the physician in sharing the treatment recommendation with the patient and/or affirming the patient's treatment preference.

Box 3.5 ○ Doctor competencies for ISDM[32]

① Establish or review the patient's preferences for information (e.g. amount, format).

② Establish or review the patient's preferences for role in decision making (e.g. risk taking, degree of involvement of self and others) and the existence/nature/degree of decisional conflict (where decisional conflict is defined as the state of uncertainty about the course of action to take).

③ Ascertain and respond to patient's ideas, concerns and expectations (e.g. about disease management options).

④ Identify choices (including ideas and information patient may have) and evaluate the research evidence in relation to the individual patient.

⑤ Present (or direct to) evidence taking into account 1 and 2 above, framing effects (i.e. where the presentation of the same information in different formats changes the decisions that people make) and helping the patient to reflect upon and assess the impact of alternative decisions *vis-à-vis* their values and lifestyles.

⑥ Make or negotiate a decision in partnership and resolve conflict.

⑦ Agree upon an action plan and complete arrangements for follow-up.

Junior doctors have been shown to focus on the disease process rather than the patient, and thus not to consider treatment options in the context of the patient's ideas, hopes and concerns.[34] Even when a menu of options is presented, the doctor may already have decided on their personal recommendation, and thus how the choices are presented is affected by this opinion.

However, there will be times when the approaches to management are completely open, with the doctor having no firm opinions as to which is preferable. Elwyn and colleagues have named this situation *clinical 'equipoise'*, defined as when the doctor admits there are two or more approaches to management and they do not have a strong view towards any of them.[35] It is at moments like these that the patient is truly involved in the decision-making process.

What do patients feel about sharing decisions in this way? In a study of women with breast cancer, important physician attributes were given as: expertise, being able to develop and maintain a personal relationship, and showing respect for patients as autonomous individuals.[36] The amount of information was not perceived to be as important as its nature and the way in which it was presented. Answering a patient's questions honestly and without hesitation was an important factor in whether the patient trusted the doctor. Although, obviously, technical proficiency was as important as the ability to communicate, we should expect our doctors to have both. The proficient surgeon known for skilful operating needs to have the ability to communicate, just as the GP with excellent communication skills needs to be able to diagnose and manage a wide range of conditions.

Sharing decisions to do nothing

With regards to management decisions, one option will always be to do nothing. This is a delicate situation if doctor and patient do not immediately agree, in what may be termed a 'wait and see' scenario. The doctor may decide a patient needs investigation or a prescription. The patient may decline either or both. Note the use of the word 'decline', a far less emotive way of describing the patient's behaviour than 'refuse'. In the shared decision-making model it is better for the doctor to know about the patient's choice to do nothing, not to make an appointment for tests, or not to have a prescription dispensed, than for the doctor to assume that the management plan is being carried out.

The other common situation is that patients present with symptoms or problems that they may initially expect to be investigated. They certainly would like an explanation for their condition and often have concerns about the possibility of underlying serious illnesses. However, the assumption that patients with unexplained symptoms pressurise doctors for symptomatic intervention has recently been challenged. In a qualitative study from Liverpool, Ring and colleagues suggest that the reason doctors intervene in this way is either because they mistake the patients' insistence on conveying the reality of their symptoms as a desire for intervention, or because doctors lack an alternative way to respond to the patients' suffering.[37] As already discussed in Chapter 2, the patient-centred approach involves the exploration and discussion of the patient's ideas, concerns and expectations. The ISDM approach moves on from this to sharing information and explanation of the symptoms. If and when the doctor decides that the symptoms are self-limiting and/or that nothing is seriously wrong, it is generally accepted that effective management of the patient avoids investigation and prescribed treatment but includes reassurance.[38] However, in the face of unexplained or psychosomatic problems, this may be more easily written than carried out in practice.

Reassuring patients is a complex task that involves the shared decision-making skills of negotiation and consensus building. It is not always enough for the doctor to state that serious disease has been excluded. Patients want to know the meaning of their symptoms. The process of recognising that certain symptoms are part of normal human experience, and do not necessarily mean illness, has been called 'normalisation'.[39]

Normalisation within the consultation draws on familiar skills. It can only be carried out to the satisfaction of the patient if an effective explanation is given by the doctor, taking into account the patient's ideas and concerns. The explanation must include an acknowledgement and validation of the patient's suffering, a tangible mechanism to explain the symptoms and a suggestion as to ways in which the patient may share in the responsibility for managing the symptoms.[40] A successful outcome is that the patient and doctor agree that nothing needs to be done at this time, i.e. a shared decision is made to do nothing.

Objections to shared decision making

Towle and her Vancouver colleague Godolphin discuss three recurring objections they have encountered in the course of their work.[41] These include: the amount of time that the ISDM process takes in consultations; doctors stating that they already involve patients in management decisions and thus do not need extra training; and the likelihood that not all patients would want to be involved in deciding on their treatment. They suggest that if ISDM does take longer it may still be more efficient in terms of health outcomes; that the evidence shows that many doctors do not involve patients; and that patients need experience in sharing and doctors need to encourage patient autonomy.

Trisha Greenhalgh,[42] an academic GP in London, and Jeremy Gambrill,[43] a cancer patient, in commentaries on ISDM have criticised the above competencies particularly in relation to the task of developing a partnership with the patient. The process of developing a partnership, suggesting a suitable doctor–patient relationship, is complex and involves several skills of its own. Moreover, such doctor–patient relationships implying continuity are difficult to develop and maintain in today's health service, particularly where many patients with complex problems are looked after by teams of doctors and health professionals in both primary and secondary care.

However, if it is accepted that ISDM is an ideal that encompasses patient-centred care, its propagation amongst doctors is worth pursuing and its inclusion in medial education worth championing, with the proviso that the effect of ISDM needs to be 'adequately defined, developed and implemented in practice and exposed to accurate means of measurement'.[44] It is important to remember that patient-centred care does not necessarily mean sharing all information and decisions; rather it means taking into account the patient's wish for information and preference for sharing decisions or not.[45] Of course, some patients will not wish to share decisions,[46] preferring the doctor to choose the management. However, it is difficult for doctors to judge which patients prefer a non-participatory role[47] and therefore it is important for the doctor to explore patient preferences, even if the patient does not wish to make the final decision.[48] Also, the doctor should not make assumptions or value judgements as to whether a particular patient wishes to share in the decision-making process. In studies of the possible implementation of shared decision making in practice, doctors have stated that such value judgements are based on intuition or instinct, the age and perceived social class of the patient, and on how the patient reacts to the doctor's advice.[49] Other factors include the nature of the patient's condition, whether acute or chronic, and the stage or maturity of the doctor–patient relationship.[50]

Patient partnership versus consumerism

In spite of the recommendations outlined above and the evidence-based reasons to move towards a partnership between doctor and patient, the director of the King's Fund in the UK wrote in the *British Medical Journal* towards the end of 1999 that 'paternalism is endemic in the NHS'.[51] In an issue devoted primarily to patient partnerships, she argued that partners work together to achieve common goals and that their relationship is based on mutual respect for each other's skills and competencies. As successful partnerships are non-hierarchical, partners share decision making and responsibility. As well as doctors receiving better training in communication skills, patients will need to be ready to take on this decision-making responsibility.

We need to make clear that patient partnership is not a form of consumerism. The defining process is that doctor and patient share decisions but they may disagree on treatment and management options. It is also possible, and likely, that certain patients may wish to pursue types of treatment that are not yet available in a particular location or are considered too expensive to be offered in comparison with a cheaper option. While it can be expressed that patients have an ethical and legal right to refuse a certain treatment, this is very different from offering patients the consumerist right to have a specific treatment that they demand.[52] There is only a finite amount of money within a health service to provide medical expertise and care, and this must be acknowledged by both doctor and patient.

Doctors have long cherished the notion of clinical freedom, defined as the right to provide whatever treatment is considered to be the best in the interest of a particular patient. However, such clinical freedom is constrained by law and available resources.[53] Doctors require considerable skill to discuss health economics with patients, particularly when certain drugs and procedures not available within the state healthcare system can possibly be paid for by patients or their health insurers. Such treatments include plastic surgery and anti-impotence drugs. State policy may also dictate whether some procedures are ethical and legal, for example the timing of induced abortion, postmenopausal fertility treatment and euthanasia.

Patient partnership does not mean that patients have the right to choose according to their wants. Doctor and patient need to discuss issues relating to patient needs. The problem is who decides between a want and a need. There is a potential conflict between patient autonomy and professional autonomy. Hopefully if the doctor feels that a patient is demanding treatment that is inappropriate, their communication skills will be such that this position may be adequately explained to the patient, who will desist from such demands. In the real world, of course, there will sometimes be a breakdown of the doctor–patient relationship resulting from this type of interaction. Ultimately it is the doctor's professional responsibility to decide on what is appropriate, and if necessary to seek help from colleagues in difficult situations. Negotiation, conflict and its resolution are discussed further in Chapter 6; doctors' confusion resulting from the consumerist view of patient involvement is discussed further in Chapter 7.

Why ISDM is important: improving 'compliance'

We know that about 50 per cent of patients with chronic diseases do not take their medication as prescribed in fully therapeutic doses.[54] In 2003, Bensing, of the Netherlands Institute of Primary Care, and colleagues defined non-compliance as the best-hidden taboo in medical encounters,[55] though research on its antecedents and ways to improve compliance has been carried out for many years. Compliance has been defined as the extent to which a patient's actual history of drug taking corresponds to the prescribed regimen.[56] That eliciting patients' worries and expectations (patient-centred approach) and giving clear, jargon-free explanations of the diagnosis and its causes improve satisfaction and compliance was documented over 30 years ago by doctors in the USA.[57] 'Adherence' is another term that has been used to describe patient behaviour.[58]

ISDM aids concordance

A group of researchers funded in part by the Department of Health Prescribing Research Initiative in the UK has focused on the first two of the four characteristics as defined by Charles et al.[31] (see Box 3.3). Their research looks at issues relating to doctor–patient communication and prescribing, in particular misunderstandings about prescriptions and patients' unvoiced agendas regarding treatment.[59] Overall they came to the conclusion that there is little evidence at present that doctors and patients do share information and views about medicines.[60] This work is part of a larger project looking at the concept of concordance, a concept that encompasses the role of both doctor and patient as regards medicine taking. The term concordance is preferred to compliance, the latter with its overtones of paternalism and 'doctor knows best'.[61] The consensus in this field is that improved communication between doctor and patient, and ISDM in the consultation, will improve concordance, leading eventually to a reduction in the number of unwanted drugs prescribed and improved patient satisfaction.[62] 'The aim of concordance is to optimise health gain from the best use of medicines, *compatible with what the patient desires and is capable of achieving*',[62] as well as reducing the prescription of inappropriate drugs. While concordance has been defined in relation to the use of medicines, it is a word that also encompasses the process of ISDM. The optimum consultation is thus a concordant one, though perhaps this is not the most elegant way of defining the outcome.

A salutary note

As previously mentioned in Chapter 1, the 2002 Commonwealth Health Fund International Health Policy Survey of Sicker Adults found that about 50 per cent of patients in the five countries surveyed felt that their regular doctor did not ask for their ideas and opinions about treatment and care (figures ranged from 47 per cent in the USA and New Zealand to 67 per cent in the UK).[63] There are many possible reasons for these figures including lack of time, pressure of work, attitudes to patient care and lack of training. However, they show that doctors should not be complacent about their consultation behaviour and that there is room for improvement.

Partnership and healing ○ *reflections*

We do want our doctors to be healers. We know they can't always heal us. But they can tell us things we need to know and that's so important. And telling us where else we can find information and help, that is so crucial when we feel desperate or at a loss. Sometimes we need to know that 'they' don't know, or don't know yet. Sometimes we need to know that we will have to bear it, the uncertainty, the fear, in the same way we will all have to bear pain and loss. Time and again, we hear stories of how doctors have done a bit of healing simply by sharing what they know, acknowledging all this and recognising how hard it is. It eases things. GPs especially can explore with us this general coping with illness and difficulty, while managing the condition and making decisions on the way. A GP colleague told me how she feels she is embarking on a journey with a patient, on diagnosis. They look together for what is needed, a true partnership.

ISDM ○ *reflections*

'Why study for nine or more years to become a GP and then ask patients what they want to do? Surely with all my knowledge and skills I am the qualified doctor and can decide the best management plan?' This is a frequent criticism of ISDM. Of course the doctor knows the medicine, but the patient knows himself or herself. How many times have I prescribed drugs that are not taken or given advice that is not heeded? A senior partner at one surgery where I worked told me that when the building was being altered a hollow tree outside the entrance was cut down. The trunk was stuffed full of prescriptions that patients had discarded within minutes of their consultations. Anecdotal perhaps but the message is true: patients do not always do what they are told. I spent a long time with one patient talking about the advantages and disadvantages of

continued over

starting on antidepressants. She agreed to give them a try but was quite honest when I saw her again. The information in the box had put her off ... too many side effects. She had flushed the pills down the toilet. It is difficult to know how much information to give. It is also difficult to share decisions. What about the patient who asks 'What would you do, doctor?' Am I being asked for my professional opinion or my personal opinion? When counselling a patient we are careful to be non-directive, so why do we feel the need to tell patients to take the pills? Some patients find it awkward to make decisions at first, but at least we can let them decide whether to be involved. Health promotion and disease prevention are about encouraging patients to take responsibility for their own health. Sharing decisions about management is a further step in this direction. I see it now as the only way to practise. But it is difficult and requires practice.

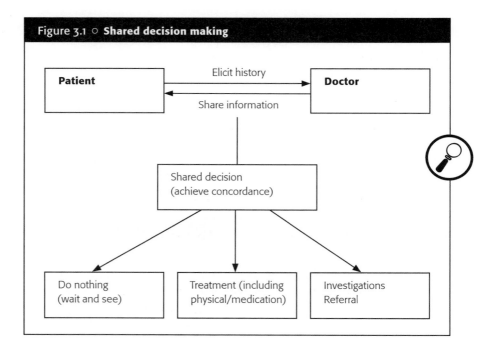

Figure 3.1 ○ **Shared decision making**

○ Summary

● Though a patient-centred approach may be used to gather information, the second half of the consultation may revert to a doctor-centred approach.

- Doctors decide how much and what information to share with patients and this information sharing may be biased because of several factors.

- Doctors often underestimate the amount of information patients wish to receive and want to spare patients from information that patients might find upsetting.

- In the informed model the physician adopts a completely neutral stance and gives the patient a range of options without expressing any preference.

- The 'informed model' has been criticised as sacrificing competence for consumerism.

- The shared decision-making model, which incorporates the notions of the patient as partner and management by negotiation, is now preferred.

- For such shared decision making to be carried out in practice the commitment of both doctor and patient to engage in the process is crucial, although the extent of involvement may vary.

REFERENCES

1 Hippocrates. *Aphorisms*. Translated by W Jones. Cambridge: Harvard University Press, 1967.

2 Fletcher C M. *Communication in Medicine*. Oxford: Nuffield Provincial Hospitals Trust, 1973.

3 Walton J, Duncan A S, Fletcher C M, Freeling P, Hawkins C, Kessel N and McCall I. *Talking with Patients, a Teaching Approach*. London: Nuffield Provincial Hospitals Trust, 1980.

4 Freidson E. *Professional Dominance*. New York: Atherton, 1970, p. 143.

5 Freidson E. *Profession of Medicine: A Study of the Sociology of Applied Knowledge*. New York: Dodd Mead, 1970, pp. 369–70.

6 Haug M and Lavin B. *Consumerism in Medicine*. London: Sage, 1983.

7 Kindelan K and Kent G. Concordance between patients' information preferences and general practitioners' perceptions. *Psychology and Health* 1987; **1**: 399–409.

8 Hingorani M, Wong T and Vafidis G. Patients' and doctors' attitudes to amount of information given after unintended injury during treatment: cross sectional, questionnaire survey. *BMJ* 1999; **318**: 640–1.

9 Burstin H, Lipsitz S R and Brennan T A. Socioeconomic status and the risk for substandard medical care. *Journal of the American Medical Association* 1992; **268**: 2383–7.

10 Levinson W, Roter D L, Mullooly J P, *et al*. Physician–patient communication. The relationship with malpractice claims among primary care physicians and surgeons. *Journal of the American Medical Association* 1997; **277**: 533–9.

11 Roter D. Which facets of communication have strong effects on outcome – a meta-analysis. In: Stewart M and Roter D (eds). *Communicating with Medical Patients*. London: Sage, 1989, pp. 183–96.

12 Hadlow J and Pitts M. The understanding of common terms by doctors, nurses and patients. *Social Science and Medicine* 1991; **32**: 193–6.

13 Stewart M, Brown J B, Weston W W, McWhinney I R, McWilliam C L and Freeman T R. *Patient-Centered Medicine. Transforming the Clinical Method*. California: Sage, 1995.

14 Levenstein J H, McCracken E C, McWhinney I R, *et al*. The patient-centred clinical method. 1. A model for the doctor–patient interaction in family medicine. *Family Practice* 1986; **3**: 24–30.

15 Horder J and Moore G T. The consultation and health outcomes. *BJGP* 1990; **40**: 442–3.

16 Szasz T S and Hollender M H. The basic model of the doctor–patient relationship. *Archives of Internal Medicine* 1956; **97**: 585.

17 Roter D L and Hall J A. *Doctors Talking with Patients/Patients Talking with Doctors*. Connecticut: Auburn House, 1992.

18 Beauchamp T and Childress J. *Principles of Biomedical Ethics*. New York: Oxford University Press, 1979.

19 Tomlinson T. The physician's influence on patient's choices. *Theoretical Medicine* 1986; **7**: 105–21.

20 Brody H. Autonomy revisited: progress in medical ethics: discussion paper. *Journal of the Royal Society of Medicine* 1985; **78**: 380–7.

21 Quill T E and Brody H. Physician recommendations and patient autonomy: finding a balance between physician power and patient choice. *Annals of Internal Medicine* 1996; **125**: 763–9.

22 Pew-Fetzer Task Force on Advancing Psychosocial Health Education. *Health Professions Education and Relationship-Centered Care: Report of the Pew-Fetzer Task Force on Advancing Psychosocial Health Education*. San Francisco: Pew Health Professions Commission, 1994.

23 Lukes S. *Power: A Radical View*. London: Macmillan, 1974.

24 Canter R. Patients and medical power. *BMJ* 2001; **323**: 414.

25 Mazur D J. Influence of the law on risk and informed consent. *BMJ* 2003; **327**: 731–4.

26 Katz J. *The Silent World of Doctor and Patient*. London and Baltimore: Johns Hopkins University Press, 1984.

27 NHS Executive. *Patient Partnership: Building a Collaborative Strategy*. Leeds: NHS Executive, 1996.

28 Edwards A, Evans R and Elwyn G. Manufactured but not imported: new direction for research in shared decision making support and skills. *Patient Education and Counseling* 2003; **50**: 33–8.

29 Towle A. *Physician and Patient Communication Skills: Competencies for Informed Shared Decision-Making* [Informed Shared Decision-Making Project]. Vancouver: University of British Columbia, 1997.

30 Elwyn G, Edwards A and Kinnersley P. Shared decision-making in primary care: the neglected second half of the consultation. *BJGP* 1999; **49**: 477–82.

31 Charles C, Gafni A and Whelan T. Shared decision-making in the medical encounter: what does it mean? (or it takes two to tango). *Social Science and Medicine* 1997; **44**: 681–92.

32 Towle A, Godolphin W and Richardson A. *Competencies for Informed Shared Decision-Making (ISDM): Report on Interviews with Physicians, Patients and Patient Educators and Focus Group Meetings with Patients.* Vancouver: University of British Columbia, 1997.

33 Lelie A. Decision-making in nephrology: shared decision making? *Patient Education and Counseling* 2000; **42**: 81–90.

34 Corke C F, Stow P J, Green D T, Agar J W and Henry M J. How doctors discuss major interventions with high risk patients: an observational study. *BMJ* 2005; **330**:182, doi:10.1136/bmj.38293.435069.DE.

35 Elwyn G, Edwards A, Kinnersley P and Grol R. Shared decision making and the concept of equipoise: defining the competences of involving patients in health care choices. *BJGP* 2000; **50**: 892–9.

36 Wright E B, Holcombe C and Salmon P. Doctors' communication of trust, care and respect in breast cancer: qualitative study. *BMJ* 2004; **328**: 864–70.

37 Ring A, Dowrick C, Humphris G and Salmon P. Do patients with unexplained physical symptoms pressurise general practitioners for somatic treatment? A qualitative study. *BMJ* 2004; **328**: 1057, doi:10.1136/bmj.38057.622639.EE.

38 Walker E A, Unutzer J and Katon W J. Understanding and caring for the distressed patient with multiple medically unexplained symptoms. *Journal of the American Board of Family Practice* 1998; **11**: 347–56.

39 Kessler D and Hamilton W. Normalisation: horrible word, useful idea. *BJGP* 2004; **54**: 163–4.

40 Dowrick C F, Ring A, Humphris G M and Salmon P. Normalisation of unexplained symptoms by general practitioners: a functional typology. *BJGP* 2004; **54**: 165–70.

41 Towle A and Godolphin W. Framework for teaching and learning informed shared decision-making. *BMJ* 1999; **319**: 766–71.

42 Greenhalgh T. Commentary: competencies for informed shared decision-making. *BMJ* 1999; **319**: 770.

43 Gambrill J. Commentary: proposals based on too many assumptions. *BMJ* 1999; **319**: 770–1.

44 Elwyn G. Shared decision making. Patient involvement in clinical practice. PhD thesis. Nijmegen, 2001, p. 11.

45 Stewart M. Towards a global definition of patient centred care. *BMJ* 2001; **322**: 444–5.

46 Guagagnoli E and Ward P. Patient participation in decision making. *Social Science and Medicine* 1998; **47**: 329–39.

47 Strull W M, Lo B and Charles G. Do patients want to participate in medical decision-making? *Journal of the American Medical Association* 1984; **252**: 2990–4.

48 Bowling A and Ebrahim S. Measuring patients' preferences for treatment and perceptions of risk. *Quality Health Care* 2001; **10 (Suppl. I)**: 2–8.

49 Thistlethwaite J E and van der Vleuten C. Informed shared decision making: views and competencies of pre-registration house officers in hospital and general practice. *Education for Primary Care* 2004; **15**: 83–92.

50 Edwards A, Elwyn G, Wood F, *et al.* Shared decision making and risk communication in practice: a qualitative study of GPs' experiences. *BJGP* 2005; **55**: 6–13.

51 Coulter A. Paternalism or partnership. *BMJ* 1999; **319**: 719–20.

52 Downie R S and Macnaughton J. *Clinical Judgement. Evidence in Practice.* Oxford: Oxford University Press, 2000.

53 Randall F. Judgement and resource management. In: Downie R S and Macnaughton J. *Clinical Judgement. Evidence in Practice.* Oxford: Oxford University Press, 2000, pp. 128–52.

54 Sackett D L and Snow J C. The magnitude of compliance and non-compliance. In: R B Haynes, Taylor W D and Sackett D L (eds). *Compliance in Health Care.* London: Johns Hopkins University Press, 1979, pp. 11–22.

55 Bensing J, van Dulmen S and Tates K. Communication in context: new directions in communication research. *Patient Education and Counseling* 2003; **50**: 27–32.

56 Urquhart J. Patient non-compliance with drug regimens: measurement, clinical correlates, economic impact. *European Heart Journal* 1996; **17 (Suppl. A)**: 8–15.

57 Korsch B M, Gozzi E K and Francis V. Gaps in doctor–patient communication. *Pediatrics* 1968; **42**: 855–71.

58 Vermeire E, Hearnshaw H, Van Royen P and Denekens J. Patient adherence to treatment: three decades of research. A comprehensive review. *Journal of Clinical Pharmacy and Therapeutics* 2001; **26**: 331–42.

59 Barry C A, Bradley C P, Britten N, Stevenson F A and Barber N. Patients' unvoiced agendas in general practice consultations: qualitative study. *BMJ* 2000; **320**: 1246–50.

60 Stevenson F A, Barry C A, Britten N, Barber N and Bradley C. Doctor–patient communication about drugs: the evidence for shared decision making. *Social Science and Medicine* 2000; **50**: 829–40.

61 Marinker M. Personal paper: writing prescriptions is easy. *BMJ* 1997; **314**: 747–8.

62 Royal Pharmaceutical Society of Great Britain. *From Compliance to Concordance. Achieving Shared Goals in Medicine Taking.* London: RPSGB, 1997.

63 Blendon R J, Schoen C, Des Roches C, Osborn R and Zapert K. Common concerns amid diverse systems: health care experiences in five countries. *Health Affairs* 2003; **22**: 106–21.

Sharing information

Evidence and risks

This chapter explores:

- the content of the information to be shared between doctor and patient • evidence-based medicine (EBM) and its role in the consultation • sharing evidence-based decisions with patients • risk communication
- decision aids • dealing with uncertainty.

'Experimental physicians ... should be able to help the sick by every means in the possession of practical medicine. What is more, with the help of the scientific spirit that guides them, they will do their part in founding experimental medicine; and that should be the most ardent wish of all physicians who want to see medicine rise out of its present state. ... I said above that compassion and blind empiricism are the prime movers of medicine; later came reflection bringing doubt, then scientific verification. This medical evolution can still be verified around us every day, for every man goes on learning, as does all humankind.'

CLAUDE BERNARD – THE FATHER OF PHYSIOLOGY[1]

The previous chapter explored the mechanisms of sharing information and making decisions: how this might be done and why it is important. This chapter discusses in more depth the content of the information to be shared and its bearing on the decision-making process.

As already described, two of the steps in the shared decision-making process are:

- transferring technical information to the patient on the treatment options, risks and probable benefits in an unbiased, clear and simple way.

- helping the patient conceptualise the weighing process of risks versus benefits and ensuring that their preferences are based on fact and not misconception.

The quantity and quality of the technical information is of paramount importance in helping the patient reach a decision about management. The information will include not only concrete evidence but also conjecture, and will almost certainly be coloured by the doctor's experience of dealing with similar cases in the past.

Discussing all the options: who decides?

The 18 July 2004 edition of the *Observer* newspaper carried a report of the case of a patient with a brain tumour.[2] The journalist and health editor, Jo Revill, wrote that the story 'gives a startling insight into the problems faced by patients who are not told about the full range of options for treatment'. The patient was advised by specialists at two different hospitals that radio-therapy was the best course of treatment. She was not informed about the option of brain surgery being offered by a London neurosurgeon but heard of it 'by chance'. She opted for surgery after being told that it carried a 5 per cent risk of leaving her disabled. So far the surgery has been a success. The patient wondered why none of her doctors had told her about this treatment and is reported as saying 'perhaps they didn't do so because it carries a risk of death and because there is little firm data yet to show whether it's better than radiotherapy, but surely that's my choice as a patient?'

Evidence-based medicine (EBM)

How do doctors decide on a management plan? What influences the choice of treatment and the options suggested to the patient? It is interesting to reflect on these questions after reading such a case or being involved in similar cases oneself. Perhaps in the case of that patient, her doctors were not aware of all the options themselves, or perhaps they judged it best to discuss only those options for which they had the evidence and risk profile. The patient was not happy and wanted to be more involved in the decisions about her own condition.

While medical science has been involved in scientific inquiry since at least the Enlightenment, it seems the move towards a more evidence-based approach to treatment has been more fashionable and yet more controver-sial for the last decade. The experience of the individual, either doctor or patient, should be correlated with results from systematic research; it is this combination of evidence and experience that ought to be discussed with the patient in order for a decision on management to be made.

A definition of EBM is:

the conscientious, explicit, and judicious use of current best evidence in making decisions about the care of individual patients. The practice of evidence based medicine means integrating individual clinical expertise with the best available external clinical evidence from systematic research. By individual clinical expertise we mean the proficiency and judgment that individual clinicians acquire through clinical experience and clinical practice. Increased expertise is reflected in many ways, but especially in more effective and efficient diagnosis and in the more thoughtful identification and compassionate use of individual patients' predicaments, rights, and preferences in making clinical decisions about their care. By best available external clinical evidence we mean clinically relevant research, often from the basic sciences of medicine, but especially from patient centred clinical research into the accuracy and precision of diagnostic tests (including the clinical examination), the power of prognostic markers, and the efficacy and safety of therapeutic, rehabilitative, and preventive regimens. External clinical evidence both invalidates previously accepted diagnostic tests and treatments and replaces them with new ones that are more powerful, more accurate, more efficacious, and safer.[3]

There would seem little contentious in the definition, especially as individual clinical expertise garnered through experience is recognised quite rightly as a prime factor in physician decision making. However, in the real world problems arise for clinicians when considering the EBM process.

Suggested steps involved in the practice of EBM are shown in Box 4.1.

Box 4.1 ○ Steps for EBM[4]

① Convert information needs into answerable questions.

② Track down the best evidence to answer these questions.

③ Critically appraise the evidence for its validity and importance.

④ Integrate this appraisal with clinical expertise and patient values to apply the results in clinical practice.

⑤ Evaluate performance.

In practice GPs do not often work in this way. Once a tentative or definitive diagnosis is made of a patient's problems, we suggest from our own experience that the doctor will base the management decision on one or more of the factors shown in Box 4.2. If there is a choice of options these may be

---

Box 4.2 ○ Factors in management decisions

○ Have always managed this condition this way.

○ Taught at medical school.

○ The article I read last week.

○ The pharmaceutical representative who fed me yesterday.

○ Something I read in the national press.

○ What the local cardiologist has started prescribing.

○ The cost.

○ Because I can remember the dose of the drug.

○ Patient's concurrent conditions and drugs.

○ The end of the week.

○ There is sound evidence as to the effectiveness of this treatment.

○ Fewer side effects.

○ My last patient did well on this.

○ My last patient had an adverse reaction to that.

○ I remember a patient with a similar story.

○ I would take this myself in similar situations.

○ The patient wants something 'natural'.

○ The patient has asked for this treatment.

○ The patient has read about this on the internet and has a printout to show me.

---

discussed with the patient adopting the shared decision-making model.

In their research on the use of explicit evidence, GPs Gabbay and le May from the University of Southampton define those collectively reinforced and internalised tacit guidelines that doctors use in everyday practice as 'mindlines'. These guidelines are based on factors similar to those in Box 4.2 and include brief reading, interactions with peers, opinion leaders, patients and pharmaceutical representatives, and the doctor's own early training and experience.[5] In this context 'tacit' means 'knowledge in practice', the informal process of experiential learning involving reflection, in contrast with explicit knowledge derived from research.

Of course, we might like to suppose that all GP treatment decisions have a sound evidence base, tacit or otherwise. We know this is not true. General practitioners often base their treatment decisions on a trial of one. If I prescribe a new drug and the patient reacts badly to it, or it doesn't work, I am less likely to prescribe it again in a hurry, whatever the journals and the drug representatives say.

However, we do expect that the newer pharmaceutical treatments we prescribe have been subjected to a rigorous research process prior to their release onto the market and that there is documented evidence about their success somewhere in the literature. Our experience of their subsequent effects may affect our choice of treatment but, in general, we do not believe that it is our role to vet drugs and chase up systematic reviews for every new product.

This trial-of-one method is consistent with the theory that doctors make diagnostic and treatment decisions based on the 'illness scripts' of patients they have seen in the past.[6] The current patient, story, symptoms and signs are run through the large database that contains all the patients who have consulted that doctor in the past. Similar cases are recalled, and, if a tentative or firm diagnosis is made, a similar treatment plan to those previous cases is chosen.

Issues relating to evidence

A major problem with clinical work is the speed with which medicine is advancing. It is easy to become out-of-date within a few months if we do not keep up with our continuing professional development. Often new ideas and refutation of old ones appear in the lay press prior to their widespread advertisement in medical journals. So sometimes we are confronted by questions that cannot be answered on the spot. Doctors need to have the knowledge and skills to search for evidence when faced with unusual cases or patients with rare conditions, or even patients with a source of information not previously accessed by the doctors themselves.

One of the prime professional attributes that medical graduates are expected to acquire during their long and arduous education is the desire for *lifelong learning*. They also need the tools to carry this out, and a healthy degree of scepticism. You cannot always believe what you read in the papers (or journals).

Published evidence may have flaws. People have vested interests in having work published. Nowadays authors of research papers have to declare any conflicting interests in their work, i.e. was their study on drug X financed by the company that manufactures X? It may be difficult to relate research data to clinical work and health services, and to find its significance for everyday practice. This has been blamed on the longstanding cultural divide between researchers, practitioners and administrators. Research, individual and institutional agendas may operate in virtual isolation.[7]

For many doctors the statistical data in papers will need to be accepted on faith and we would hope that it has been scrutinised carefully by reviewers. But how often do we read the whole study at the primary source? By the time we come to assess the evidence it may have passed through several commentaries and paraphrasing. Editorials are often a good method of assimilating the message of one or more pieces of work. However, even these are flawed. There is certainly a bias towards producing and publishing positive results.[8] However, this is likely to change following a directive from the editors of medical journals that all clinical trials must be registered so that both negative and positive results are in the public domain.[9]

To overcome possible bias, clinicians may turn to *systematic reviews*. These reviews take some of the hard work out of assessing evidence by presenting, criticising and formulating as much of the available evidence as possible on a particular topic. Systematic reviews have been defined as scientific investigations that include a synthesis of the results of multiple primary investigations by using strategies that limit bias and random error.[10] Systematic reviews may be quantitative or qualitative. Meta-analyses are quantitative reviews that use statistical methods to combine the results of two or more studies. Qualitative reviews summarise primary studies without statistically combining them.[8] However, GPs may still criticise published evidence as not being relevant to their own practice. Level I in the hierarchy of evidence (Table 4.1),[11] representing the most robust evidence, is based on the results from randomised controlled trials. Much of the data presented in such trials arises from trials on a population dissimilar to that found in the community. The patients excluded from the trial may be characteristic of the patient sitting in the surgery chair.

Table 4.1 ○ **The hierarchy of evidence**[11]

Level	Type of evidence
I	Strong evidence from at least one systematic review of multiple, well-designed, randomised controlled trials
II	Strong evidence from at least one properly designed, randomised controlled trial of appropriate size
III	Evidence from well-designed trials without randomisation, single-group pre-post, cohort, time series or matched case-control studies
IV	Evidence from well-designed, non-experimental studies from more than one centre or research group
V	Opinions of respected authorities, based on clinical evidence, descriptive studies or reports of expert committees

SOURCE: Muir Gray JA. *Evidence-Based Healthcare*. Edinburgh: Churchill Livingstone, 1997.

Evidence also becomes out-of-date very quickly. Treatments that were the fashion and supposedly effective just a few years ago may now seem outdated or frankly dangerous. This can be due to newer, improved treatments arriving in the pharmacopoeia or to new evidence being produced, in part due to greater numbers of patients taking a treatment since the clinical trials that helped launch it on the market. Recent examples of major swings in opinion relating to treatment are those of hormone replacement therapy (HRT) and the use of beta-blockers in heart failure. HRT was regarded by many as an effective treatment for the management of the menopause, and a safe therapy for the prevention of ischaemic heart disease. How times change! The number of women starting HRT has dropped markedly [12] and the dangers of the drug have been published extensively. At one time beta-blockers were contraindicated in patients with heart failure; now these relatively old drugs have been recommended as one of several to be considered for this condition.[13] Recall of once lauded therapies, such as refecocoxib (Vioxx) in 2004, due to ongoing trials after the drug gains a licence, may make GPs wary of prescribing newer treatments too quickly.

Textbooks are out-of-date almost as soon as they are printed. Journals fare better in their impact but even then some of the articles may have been written several months ago. Check the date of submission if it is printed with a paper for evidence of this fact. The medium that keeps pace best with change is the World Wide Web via the internet. The problem here though is that much of the information on the Web is not vetted or checked for accuracy; it is not all peer-reviewed. Yet it is the place where many of our patients will be checking on their treatments and weighing up their options (see Chapter 10 for more on this).

Some sources of evidence are shown in Box 4.3. The electronic databases may be accessed in surgeries. Familiarity with the layout and search capabilities of these speeds up the process of accessing evidence but discrimination is still required when considering the uses to which such evidence should be put. Evidence is only part of the clinical decision-making process.[14] Doctors must use clinical expertise to evaluate an individual patient's circumstances.

Guidelines in practice

In spite of the limitations of EBM, a survey of GPs carried out a few years ago found that respondents mainly welcomed EBM and agreed that its practice improves patient care. However, they had a low level of awareness of how to extract evidence from journals, review publications and databases,

Box 4.3 ○ **Easily accessible sources of evidence**

○ Peer-referenced journals – many of these are now accessible on-line: http://bmj.bmjjournals.com/ has a useful search engine (there is a charge for this service).

○ *British National Formulary.*

○ *Clinical Evidence* from BMJ Publishing: a compendium of summaries of the best available evidence about what works and what doesn't work, updated regularly.[15]

○ The internet: numerous medical sites including those for all the royal colleges.

○ Medline and Ovid: these are search engines available on-line and containing references from over 3600 peer-reference journals.

○ Cochrane library: www.cochrane.co.uk is a database of systematic reviews.

and, even if aware, many did not use them. The major perceived barrier to practising EBM was lack of personal time. These GPs thought that the most appropriate way to move towards evidence-based general practice was by using evidence-based guidelines or proposals developed by colleagues.[16] Guidelines are defined as systematically developed statements to assist practitioner and patient decisions about appropriate health care in specific clinical circumstances.[17] They are usually compiled by expert groups and their use may be checked by audit activities.[7]

While skills in searching for evidence may have increased, it is likely that most GPs would still prefer a method of using evidence that takes the least amount of time for the maximum gain. However, GPs deal with many different problems every day in short consultations and are unlikely to remember every guideline that is produced. Regular practice meetings are needed to discuss implementation of relevant guidelines, and their use reinforced by strategies such as computerised reminders, having regularly revised loose-leaf practice manuals in each consulting room and providing educational activities within the practice.[18] While guidelines that are developed by the clinicians who are likely to use them are more successful (as this development generates a sense of local ownership),[19] researching and writing the guidelines is time consuming.

Sharing evidence-based decisions with patients

On the whole patients trust their doctors unless that trust has been lost through bad practice or poor treatment outcomes. When a doctor discusses treatment options with patients, most patients, we can assume, will trust the doctor to offer them choices based on knowledge and training, choices that work. Patients may not use the word evidence but they certainly expect their doctors to know what they are talking about. However, patients will accept explanations and treatments that have not been evaluated within the scientific model that we practise. Complementary and alternative medicine is very popular in the UK, much of which has no research backing. Many patients' health belief systems persuade them that natural remedies are safer than orthodox treatments. While some people are sceptical about things they read in the paper, articles and advertising features on the internet are often taken as the truth. All these factors can lead to complex discussions between doctor and patient if the doctor wishes the patient to be fully informed of the facts and to understand some of the issues relating to evidence and proof of efficacy.

Patients may challenge the doctor's opinion or suggest alternative management plans. This may be perceived as threatening behaviour, undermining the doctor's knowledge and skills. The doctor needs exceptional communication and negotiation skills to manage these situations for the best outcome for both doctor and patient (see Chapter 6 for more on this). Doctors also need to recognise that some patients with rare conditions will have more information about their illnesses than their treating physician. Expert patients are increasingly being recognised as a resource in education and training,[20] but they also need to access health care.

Sharing information: issues of quality and quantity

Here you go, said the doctor, scribbling me a prescription; I think what you need is some antidepressants. I was depressed, so I knew it made a kind of sense. Twenty-four hours later, I found I couldn't read; print blurred before my eyes. I went to the university library and tried to look up the side effects of the drug, but I was labouring under the obvious handicap. In those days (1972), pills didn't come with a patient information leaflet. Your doctor had all the information you needed, and whether you could get it depended on whether you had pull, face and cunning. I have none of these.

HILARY MANTEL[21]

General practitioners cannot be expected to know about every condition and treatment option in depth. Therefore it is important that practices have access to information in other formats that can be given to patients. Printed leaflets, audiotapes, videos and CD-ROMs are available and may be used as sources of information and prompts for patients to use in discussion with their doctors. They are more likely to increase patients' understanding if they are structured, tailored to the individual and/or interactive.[22] The information contained in such materials should of course be vetted for accuracy by the doctor who is handing them out. They should also be scrutinised for readability and usefulness. This may be difficult if non-English material is used.

Coulter and colleagues have identified the sorts of information that patients require in order to be involved in decisions about health care (Box 4.4).[23] In this study for the King's Fund on sources of information for patients, the researchers noticed an assumption on the part of many information producers that patients do not want to know about side effects. However, patients were adamant that they did want to see the full picture, as long as it was presented in a non-alarmist fashion. Patients prefer information that is balanced and includes a careful and honest assessment of the advantages and disadvantages of treatment. They do not want false reassurance if outcome probabilities are unknown because relevant research has not been carried out.[23]

Box 4.4 ○ Information needs of patients [23]

- ○ Understanding what is wrong.
- ○ A realistic idea of prognosis.
- ○ How to make the most of consultations.
- ○ The processes and likely outcomes of possible tests and treatments.
- ○ How to assist in self-care.
- ○ Available services and sources of help.
- ○ Reassurance and help to cope.
- ○ Helping others understand.
- ○ Legitimising seeking help and their concerns.
- ○ How to prevent further illness.
- ○ How to identify further information and self-help groups.
- ○ How to identify the 'best' healthcare providers.

Doctors who know the kinds of questions that patients would like to ask are in a position to provide this information without being prompted (Box 4.5). In relation to drug treatment they wish to know about four essential aspects of their medicine (Box 4.6).[24] Obviously, anxious patients may not remember all the queries they have. Patients often have difficulty asking questions because they feel intimidated and are concerned about using the doctor's time.[25] They are also not likely to remember all the information doctors impart, perhaps forgetting as much as 80 per cent of what is discussed in the consultation.[26] Therefore follow-up appointments are important as well as the materials discussed above.

Box 4.5 ○ The questions patients would like to ask

What is wrong with me?	Why has this happened?
Why has it happened now?	Does it run in families?
Do other people have this problem?	Will my children get it?
What can I do to help myself?	Is it my fault?
What is likely to happen to me?	Will I get better?
Will I get worse?	What are these tests for?
Will they hurt?	When will I get the results?
Should I see a specialist?	Why am I seeing a specialist?
How long will it take?	What will happen at the hospital?
Will it be quicker if I pay?	Do I have to go to the local hospital?
Is there any treatment for this?	Is there a choice of treatment?
Will this treatment work?	How long will it take?
What are the side effects?	What happens if I don't take it?
Will this drug make me depressed?	Will it make me impotent?
Is the drug addictive?	Is there a more natural treatment?
How long do I have to take it for?	Which treatment is the best?
Is there a cure?	Will there ever be a cure?
What should I tell my family?	What will you tell my family?
Where can I get more information?	Do I have a choice in what happens next?

Box 4.6 ○ Essential information about drugs[24]

○ Side effects.

○ What it does and what it's for.

○ Do's and don'ts.

○ How to take it.

Differences in decision support

The options available to patients for any particular condition have been labelled either 'effective' or 'preference sensitive'.[27] Effective options are those that include management choices where guidelines or a standard of care have been defined. The doctor may then legitimately feel that counselling should be directive and the doctor's recommendation outlined. Examples of effective options are monitoring blood lipids in patients with diabetes, the use of aspirin in the secondary prevention of ischaemic heart disease and the health risks of smoking. Preference-sensitive options are those for which there is no clear evidence to recommend one option above another. Counselling should thus be non-directive. How the patient chooses will depend on the value they put on the possible benefits compared to any possible harm. The patient also has to be aware of the scientific uncertainties. Examples of preference-sensitive options at present include screening for prostate cancer, the treatment of early-stage breast cancer and the management of back pain. Of course, as new evidence is emerging constantly preference-sensitive options may become effective options in time.

Discussing risk: risk communication

○ **Risk** *the possibility of suffering harm or loss; danger; the chances that a hazard will give rise to harm.*

Discussing and negotiating a management plan should involve enabling patients to understand risk: risk of the condition, risk of treatment, risk of non-treatment, risk to other people, etc. Risk may be defined at a very simplistic level. For example, a doctor may say 'If you do not use contraception you are likely to get pregnant.' This statement is true and most women would understand and agree with it. They may not take the advice, but that is another facet of risk behaviour. Patients are influenced by a number of factors when listening to information about risk (Box 4.7).[28] The trust patients have for their doctors is thus of paramount importance in the process of risk communication. However, paradoxically, patients will often believe information they read in the papers at the expense of information gained from health professionals. A recent example of this has been the reluctance of patients to have their children immunised with the MMR vaccine.

Box 4.7 ○ Influences on response to information about risk[28]

○ The extent to which the source of information is trusted.

○ The relevance of the information for everyday life and decision making.

○ The relation to other perceived risks.

○ The fit with previous knowledge and experience.

○ The difficulty and importance of the choices and decisions.

Once we start defining risk in terms of probabilities with numbers attached, the process becomes more complex. Bias and errors creep into the figures (Table 4.2).[29]

Table 4.2 ○ **Common errors relating to risk[29]**

Error	Definition
Miscalibration bias	Overestimation of the level and accuracy of one's knowledge
Compression bias	Tendency to overestimate small risks and underestimate large ones
Availability bias	Overestimation of notorious risks
Optimism–pessimism bias	Tendency of patients to believe that they are less at risk of an adverse outcome than people similar to them

Risk communication is the open, two-way exchange of information and opinion about risk, which should lead to better understanding and better decisions about clinical management.[30] Note that this definition involves sharing information, rather than the notion that information is communicated only from clinician to patient. The patient is asked to discuss the acceptability of the risk that is under scrutiny. This exchange of information and opinion is important if treatment decisions are to reflect the attitudes to risk of the patients who will live with the outcomes.[31]

Patients understand different methods of presenting risk to varying extents.[32] As with all information that is imparted by a doctor, the language may be misunderstood or misinterpreted. Risk language is often ambiguous. What is meant by 'likely'? 'Common' is difficult to quantify, while 'rare' is context specific. If a patient knows someone with a rare condition, they have a different picture of its probability from other people. As medical students in tertiary hospitals we often saw 'rare' conditions, but as general practitioners we are unlikely to see another such case in our careers.

Risk is generally defined in terms of numerical odds or probabilities, yet research has shown that patients find such terms difficult to understand, and that their understanding is affected by their age, educational level, health status and recent experience of illness.[33] Kenneth Calman, the UK's Chief Medical Officer from 1991 to 1998, has classified a language of risk to help overcome the public's confusion in relation to common terms that are often used in conflicting ways.[34] He and Royston of the NHS Executive have also suggested combining standardised terms and specified frequencies, and displaying these on a risk scale with easily understandable descriptions[35] (Table 4.3).

Table 4.3 ○ **Community risk scale**[35]

Risk	Risk magnitude	Risk description (unit in which one adverse event would be expected)	Example (based on number of deaths in Britain per year)
1 in 1	10	Person	
1 in 10	9	Family	
1 in 100	8	Street	Any cause
1 in 1000	7	Village	Any cause, age 40
1 in 10,000	6	Small town	Road accident
1 in 100,000	5	Large town	Murder
1 in 1,000,000	4	City	Oral contraceptives
1 in 10,000,000	3	Province or country	Lightning
1 in 100,000,000	2	Large country	Measles
1 in 1,000,000,000	1	Continent	

SOURCE: Calman K and Royston G. Risk language and dialects. *BMJ* 1997; **315**: 941.

Communicating risk in this way assumes that patients will want to make rational decisions, but patients' health beliefs and personal experiences may lead them to choices that seem irrational to doctors.[36] Risk evidence rarely includes psychosocial outcomes, although these are important to individual patients.[37] Short-term gain is often a more powerful motivator than long-term benefits.[38] This type of balancing of risks is a fundamental process in human behaviour. People take risks with their health for immediate pleasure, for example club culture and Ecstasy use, extreme sports and binge drinking of alcohol. Thus shared decision making and its outcome, in terms of an individual patient's choice, are unpredictable. Patients may also change their minds between one consultation and the next. Doctors must be wary of making assumptions, however well they think they know their patients.

Decisions aids

○ **Decision aid** *interventions to help people make deliberative choices from healthcare options by providing information relevant to a person's health status.*[39]

Decision aids are support material that facilitate decision making. They may be used before, during or after consultations depending on when it is the optimum time to offer such support.[40] A good decision aid is one that bases risk on individual data, such as the Framingham equation for cardiovascular and cerebrovascular disease,[41] and the Dundee scales.[42] The recent availability of internet-based risk calculators allows doctors and patients to generate tailored risk information based on personal factors.[43]

The Cochrane Collaboration review team have described and registered more than 400 decision aids for patients (available on the internet at www.ohri.ca/decisionaid).[44] The aids are available in different formats including leaflets, videos, audiotapes and workbooks, as well as Web-based applications. These aids facilitate decision making by describing choices and possible outcomes. Many are personalised in that they rely on a patient's input of data to clarify individual risk. Some are also based on psychological theories of decision making and aim to help the cognitive processes that people use on information in order to make decisions. They are different from the materials mentioned earlier that just give facts.

Decision aids improve the decision-making process by increasing patients' knowledge of options, creating realistic personal expectations of outcomes and improving the match between choices and patients' values.[45] Overall they reduce the number of patients who are uncertain about what to do, but there are still many questions relating to their use in consultations and their impact on patient satisfaction and physical outcomes.[39]

Coping with uncertainty: doctors

When considering evidence, risk and choice, one of the important attributes both doctors and patients need is the ability to cope with uncertainty. Of course, life is never certain but this is not necessarily something we think about as we go about our daily lives. As Professor Katz of Yale University writes:

> It is a fact of life that human beings find it difficult to maintain a consistent, self-conscious appreciation of the extent to which uncertainty accompanies them on their daily rounds and to integrate that uncertainty with whatever certainties inform their conduct. Physicians are not exempt from this human proclivity. They will acknowledge medicine's uncertainty once its presence is forced into conscious awareness yet at the same time will continue to conduct their practice as if uncertainty did not exist.[46]

This lack of admitting to uncertainty is part of the paternalistic process. Katz relates the story of a surgeon with whom he had a discussion about the various treatments for breast cancer. The surgeon spoke of the uncertainties inherent in such treatment. However, this same surgeon said that when he consults with patients he mentions only the necessity of having an operation without indicating that any alternatives exist. He does this because he believes that patients cannot understand or tolerate an exploration of the uncertainties of treatment. Katz labels this as a problem of moving from theory to practice.[46] In theory while doctors may acknowledge uncertainty, in clinical practice they may appear omniscient and convinced of a certain management path. Yet doctors' uncertainty with regard to weighing the strength and significance of evidence may explain some of the variation seen in clinical practice.[47]

Medical education in the last decade, particularly general practice training, has emphasised the need for doctors to be able to deal with uncertainty. However, there is evidence that doctors are still not adequately trained to cope with uncertainty in practice.[48] If we are better equipped, it is unlikely that we want to show our patients our uncertainty. Yet, discussing lack of evidence, informing patients of the conflicts between experts as to what constitutes best practice and admitting that we do not always know which option is best, are all part of the shared decision-making process.

Of course, a doctor may be uncertain of facts and outcomes due to individual lack of medical knowledge in that field. Knowing what you don't know is important. Admitting that you don't know is often hard but easier in the long run. In our experience older doctors are less likely to be embarrassed at looking things up than junior doctors. After all, memory is not so good in later life and all those drug names and doses are difficult to remember.

Uncertainty is also a feature of many consultations before the management stage is reached. There may be uncertainty as to the diagnosis and the nature of the patient's problem. Dealing with medically unexplained symptoms is considered further in Chapter 5. One way for GPs to understand uncertainty and also unpredictability within consultations is to describe such consultations as 'complex' systems. *Complexity theory* looks at the interactions between components of a system, recognising that the system as a whole cannot be fully understood only by analysing such components and that complex systems cannot be adequately described by means of a simple theory.[49] Proponents of applying complexity theory to consultations suggest that this will help doctors to take risks within consultations and share their uncertainty with patients, leading to potentially different/better outcomes.[50]

Coping with uncertainty: patients

Even though patients may receive full and easily assimilated information from a skilled and patient-centred doctor they may still find it difficult to choose or make a decision. They may be struck by what has been called decisional conflict.[51] When we communicate our uncertainties to patients, they also have to learn to live with these. Maybe this is why paternalistic doctors act as they do. They hate to see their patient-children grappling with choice and discomfort. Patients are not trained to understand the complexity of medical evidence. They may wish the doctor to be more prescriptive. This is why decisions should be shared. Patients should not feel they are on their own when confronting choice. Doctors should help patients to clarify their priorities and values, and weigh up outcomes for the individual based on the patient's personal circumstances.

While a key communication objective may be the reduction of uncertainty,[52] helping patients to know what to expect, to remove it entirely is not always possible. Or at least this may be impossible during a single consultation. A woman with a breast lump who is referred for investigation has to live with uncertainty and the attendant anxiety regarding diagnosis until the tests are complete. How often do we hear medical students and junior doctors telling patients not to worry while the patients are waiting for their results? Of course you are going to worry if you have a breast lump or chest pain or abnormal bleeding until you know what is wrong.

EBM ○ *reflections*

I want the best for my patients; I want to help them and to heal them. That is my vocation as a doctor. But of course often I cannot heal. I am aware with many of my regular patients that I am a powerful and knowledgeable person in their lives. It is up to me to ensure that I keep up-to-date with medical knowledge and the evidence for it, and that I can explain treatment options in terms that my patients understand. This is very difficult. There is little time in the day to digest all the journals and new discoveries that are being made. And indeed how relevant are they all to my practice? Moreover I am often restricted in the options I can really offer by financial concerns and the availability of certain treatments in my locality. It is not simple. At present I do not use Web-based decision aids in my practice apart from those that can be easily accessed during consultations such as ischaemic heart disease (IHD) risk calculators. And while I give patients leaflets to read and time to think about decisions by arranging timely follow-up appointments, I have not yet advised them to complete a decision aid on-line and return with it. However, I think this is the next logical step in the shared decision-making process and I will be exploring the use of such aids in the near future.

Evidence, risk taking and risk communication ○ *reflections*

I've been struck, in our educational and research work with patients with long-term conditions, how much risk taking they are doing, day by day. They juggle having as normal a life as possible, say, with following, or not, a regime. They work out what seems to be best for them. But they often don't tell their doctors about it, keen to be 'good patients' and keep their doctors on side. So everyone is talking in the consultation without reference to some real evidence from experience, let alone the science. GPs seem to be in the best position to support patients to come clean about their risks and help them make good decisions.

○ **Summary**

- The quantity and quality of the technical information given to patients is of paramount importance in helping the patient reach a decision about management.

- The experience of the individual, either doctor or patient, should be correlated with results from systematic research; it is these results that ought to be discussed with the patient in order for a decision on management to be made.

- In practice we do not always think about the evidence.

- Evidence also becomes out-of-date very quickly.

- Systematic reviews take some of the hard work out of assessing evidence by presenting, criticising and formulating as much of the available evidence as possible on a particular topic.

- Guidelines are systematically developed statements to assist practitioner and patient decisions about appropriate health care in specific clinical circumstances.

- Patients prefer information that is balanced and includes a careful and honest assessment of the advantages and disadvantages of treatment.

- Patients are not likely to remember all the information doctors impart.

- Discussing and negotiating a management plan should involve enabling patients to understand risk.

- Risk communication is the open, two-way exchange of information and opinion about risk, which should lead to better understanding and better decisions about clinical management.

- A good decision aid is one that bases risk on individual data.

- Decision aids improve the decision-making process by increasing patients' knowledge of options, creating realistic personal expectations.

- Doctors and patients have to live with uncertainty.

REFERENCES

1 Bernard C. *An Introduction to the Study of Experimental Medicine*. New York: Dover Publications, 1957 [first published in 1865], pp. 212–13.

2 Revill J. Brain tumour mum awakes to a new life. *Observer*, 18 July 2004, p. 8.

3 Sackett D L, Rosenberg W M C, Muir Gray J A, Haynes R B and Richardson W S. Evidence based medicine: what it is and what it isn't. *BMJ* 1996; **312**: 71–2.

4 Straus S E and McAllister F A. Evidence-based medicine: a commentary on common criticisms. *Canadian Medical Association Journal* 2000; **163**: 837–41.

5 Gabbay J and le May A. Evidence based guidelines or collectively constructed 'mindlines'? Ethnographic study of knowledge management in primary care. *BMJ* 2004; **329**: 1488–92.

6 Schmidt H G, Norman G R and Boshuizen H P A. A cognitive perspective on medical expertise: theory and implications. *Academic Medicine* 1990; **65**: 611–21.

7 Haines A and Jones R. Implementing findings of research. *BMJ* 1994; **308**: 1488–92.

8 Muir Gray J A. Evidence-based medicine for professionals. In: Edwards A and Elwyn G. *Evidence-Based Patient Choice*. Oxford: Oxford University Press, 2001, pp. 19–33.

9 Abbasi K. Compulsory registration of all clinical trials. *BMJ* 2004; **329**: 637–8.

10 Cook D J, Mulrow C D and Haynes B R. Systematic reviews: synthesis of best evidence for clinical decisions. *Annals of Internal Medicine* 1997; **126**: 376–80.

11 Muir Gray J A. *Evidence-Based Healthcare*. Edinburgh: Churchill Livingstone, 1997.

12 Lawton B, Rose S, McLeod D and Dowell A. Changes in use of hormone replacement therapy after the report from the Women's Health Initiative: cross sectional survey of users. *BMJ* 2003; **327**: 845–6.

13 Avezum A, Tsuyuki R T, Pogue J, *et al*. Beta-blocker therapy for congestive heart failure: a systematic overview and critical appraisal of the published trials. *Canadian Journal of Cardiology* 1998; **14**: 1045–53.

14 Shaughnessy A F, Slawson D C and Becker L. Clinical jazz: harmonising clinical experience and evidence-based medicine. *Journal of Family Practice* 1998; **47**: 425–8.

15 Barton S. Using clinical evidence. *BMJ* 2001; **322**: 503–4.

16 McColl A, Smith E, White P and Field J. General practitioners' perceptions of the route to evidence based medicine: a questionnaire survey. *BMJ* 1998; **316**: 361–5.

17 Institute of Medicine. *Clinical Practice Guidelines: Directions for a New Program*. Washington, D.C.: National Academy Press, 1990.

18 Lipman T and Price D. Decision making, evidence, audit and education: case study of antibiotic prescribing in general practice. *BMJ* 2000; **320**: 1114–18.

19 Grimshaw J M and Russell I T. Effect of clinical guidelines on medical practice: a systematic review of rigorous evaluations. *Lancet* 1993; **342**: 1317–22.

20 Department of Health. *The Expert Patient: A New Approach to Chronic Disease Management for the 21st Century*. London: DoH, 2001.

21 Mantel H. *Giving up the Ghost. A Memoir*. London: Harper Perennial, 2004, p. 171.

22 Trevena L J, Davey H M, Barratt A, *et al.* A systematic review on communicating with patients about evidence. *Journal of Evaluation of Clinical Practice* 2006; **12** (**1**): 13–23, doi: 10.1111/j.1365-2753.2005.00596.x.

23 Coulter A, Entwistle V and Gilbert D. Sharing decisions with patients: is the information good enough? *BMJ* 1999; **318**: 318–22.

24 Dickinson D and Raynor D K T. Ask the patients – they may want to know more than you think. *BMJ* 2003; **327**: 861.

25 Towle A, Godolphin W, Manklow J and Wiesinger H. Patient perceptions that limit a community-based intervention to promote participation. *Patient Education and Counselling* 2003; **50**: 231–3.

26 Kessels R P C. Patients' memory for medical information. *Journal of the Royal Society of Medicine* 2003; **96**: 219–22.

27 O'Connor A, Légaré F and Stacey D. Risk communication in practice: the contribution of decision aids. *BMJ* 2003; **327**: 736–40.

28 Alaszewski A and Horlick-Jones T. How can doctors communicate information about risk more effectively? *BMJ* 2003; **327**: 728–31.

29 Bogardus S T, Holmboe E and Jeskel J F. Perils, pitfalls and possibilities in talking about medical risks. *Journal of the American Medical Association* 1999; **281**: 1037–41.

30 Edwards A G K, Hood K, Matthews E J, Russell D, Russell I T, Barker J, *et al*. The effectiveness of one-to-one risk communication interventions in health care: a systematic review. *Medical Decision Making* 2000; **20**: 290–7.

31 Edwards A, Elwyn G and Muller A. Explaining risks: turning numerical data into meaningful pictures. *BMJ* 2002; **324**: 827–30.

32 Say R E and Thomson R. The importance of patient preferences in treatment decisions – challenges for doctors. *BMJ* 2003; **327**: 542–5.

33 Mazur D J and Merz J F. Patients' interpretations of verbal expressions of probability – implications for securing informed consent to medical interventions. *Behavioural Sciences and the Law* 1994; **12**: 417–26.

34 Calman K C. Cancer: science and society and the communication of risk. *BMJ* 1996; **313**: 799–803.

35 Calman K and Royston G. Risk language and dialects. *BMJ* 1997; **315**: 939–42.

36 Thornton H. Patients' understanding of risk. *BMJ* 2003; **327**: 693–4.

37 Godolphin W. The role of risk communication in shared decision making. *BMJ* 2003; **327**: 692–3.

38 Tversky A and Kahnemann D. The framing of decisions and the psychology of choice. *Science* 1981; **211**: 453–8.

39 O'Connor A M, Stacey D, Entwistle V, Llewellyn-Thomas H, Rovner D, Holmes-Rovner M, *et al*. Decision aids for people facing health treatment or screening decisions. *BMJ* 1999; **319**: 731–4.

40 Edwards A, Evans R and Elwyn G. Manufactured but not imported: new directions for research in shared decision making support and skills. *Patient Education and Counseling* 2003; **50**: 33–8.

41 Wolf P A, D'Agostino R B, Belanger A J and Kannel W B. Probability of stroke: a risk profile from the Framingham study. *Stroke* 1991; **22**: 312–18.

42 Tunstall-Pedoe H. The Dundee coronary risk-disk for management of change in risk factors. *BMJ* 1991; **303**: 744–7.

43 Woloshin S, Schwartz LM and Ellner A. Making sense of risk information on the web. *BMJ* 2003; **327**: 695–6.

44 O'Connor AM, Stacey D, Entwistle V, Llewellyn-Thomas H, Rovner D, Holmes-Rovner M, *et al.* Decision aids for people facing health treatment or screening decisions. *Cochrane Database of Systematic Reviews* 2003; **2**: CD 001431.

45 O'Connor A and Edwards A. How do you develop and evaluate a decision aid? In: Edwards A and Elwyn G. *Evidence-Based Patient Choice*. Oxford: Oxford University Press, 2001, pp. 220–42.

46 Katz J. *The Silent World of Doctor and Patient*. London and Baltimore: Johns Hopkins University Press, 1984, p. 166.

47 McNeil BJ. Hidden barriers to improvement in the quality of care. *New England Journal of Medicine* 2001; **354**: 1612–20.

48 Djulbegovic B. Lifting the fog of uncertainty from the practice of medicine. *BMJ* 2004; **329**: 1419–20.

49 Cilliers P. *Complexity and Postmodernism*. London: Routledge, 1998.

50 Innes A D, Campion P D and Griffiths F E. Complex consultations and the 'edge of chaos'. *BJGP* 2005; **55**: 47–52.

51 O'Connor AM. Validation of a decisional conflict scale. *Medical Decision Making* 1995; **15**: 25–30.

52 Hargie C T C and Tourish D. Relational communication. In: Hargie O D W (ed.). *The Handbook of Communication Skills*. Second edition. London: Routledge, 1997, pp. 358–82.

Consultation skills techniques and strategies in more depth

This chapter discusses in more depth some of the skills and techniques mentioned in the previous chapter, as well as introducing some new topics. Where appropriate and relevant we provide research evidence to illuminate these.

This chapter explores:

- explaining ● helping patients to help themselves ● negotiation and resolving conflict ● a further look at empathy ● interacting with patients with medically unexplained/multiple symptoms ● dealing with challenging situations ● patients with disabilities ● breaking bad news ● motivational interviewing ● coping with aggression ● neuro-linguistic programming (NLP).

'Empathy consists of feeling. It involves the inner experience of feeling oneself to be similar to or nearly identical with the other person. There is an important distinction between simple empathy and the use of empathy as a technical and specialized cognitive technique. Both simple or raw empathy and empathy as the tool of the scientist are capable of yielding objective information not attainable through ordinary rational and intellectual techniques. When empathy is used in a professional way, it becomes more consistently effective, more versatile and more penetrating. With discipline, empathy, or 'empathic understanding' becomes a fully reputable scientific technique.'

RL Katz[1]

Every general practice consultation is a challenge in some way. There are techniques and strategies to deal with such challenges. Many GPs learn these through trial and error, and by experience. Some are learnt in more formal settings. There is an evidence base for many of them that justifies their use to improve outcomes. It is important, however, to realise that theory is all very well but that practical application in everyday practice is what makes evidence relevant.

Explaining

Once a problem has been identified, the doctor will be in the position of explaining a diagnosis, the reason for investigations and/or choices of management plans.

○ **Explaining** *to make plain or comprehensible; to define or expound; to offer reasons for or a cause of, to justify; to offer reasons for the actions, beliefs or remarks of oneself.*

The definitions of the word 'explaining' make interesting reading as they include aims of doctors when sharing information with patients. In Chapter 4 we discussed sharing information and the type of information that patients want and require to make decisions. This information may need to be explained; it may in its original form be unintelligible to the patient. Sharing information by the doctor may include explanation of the meaning and causes of symptoms, reasons why they have occurred and justification of any suggested treatment options. Sharing information by the patient occurs when they are invited to offer reasons for their behaviour (ideas). Patient and doctor explore and explain each other's health beliefs.

Explaining has been divided into three main types by educationalists,[2] which may be thought of in a consultation context according to the sorts of questions patients ask (Table 5.1).

Why is this important? In cases where patients may find it difficult to express their concerns or remember their questions, doctors may find it helpful to explain to patients in these three domains. In brief, for example, a patient may be wondering: what has happened to me? How did it happen? Why did it happen? Or: what are the available treatments? How do they work? Why should I choose this one?

This process may be likened to education. The doctor is a teacher helping patients understand their problems. As in any form of education the explainer must consider the existing knowledge and beliefs of the patient. To understand and assimilate new facts a person must be able to mesh the new knowledge with what they already know about the topic.[3] It is easy for doctors to assume prior knowledge. Even if we do not resort to jargon we may offer explanations far removed from a patient's own worldview. Doctors and patients use the same words but with different meanings. For example, game shows on television often include questions about the human body. Sometimes contestants are asked to put internal organs in their correct place on an anatomical figure. The stomach is often equated with the whole of the abdomen.

Table 5.1 ○ **Types of explaining**

Type of explaining	Examples of questions	Purpose
Interpretive	What?	Interpretation or clarification
	What is happening to me?	
	What is causing this rash?	
	What effects does high blood pressure have?	
	What is a heart attack?	
Descriptive	How?	Description of process, structure, procedures
	How does my liver work?	
	How do these pills have an effect on my depression?	
	How do I know I can trust you?	
Reason giving	Why?	Reasons based on principles, motives, values
	Why is this happening to me?	
	Why did I have a heart attack?	
	Why did my sister die?	
	Why should I take these pills?	

The purpose of an explanation is that the patient understands. This will help them in any decision-making process. It is an important task of the doctor's to check that understanding. Asking 'Do you understand?' is not the best method. Asking if the patient has any questions is often unhelpful. The patient should be encouraged to say what has been understood in their own words. How often do we do this in practice? A patient's lack of understanding may not be apparent until decisions about treatment are necessary. Then the whole explaining process may need to be repeated. Strategies and skills for explaining are shown in Box 5.1.

Box 5.1 ○ **Explaining skills and strategies**

○ Adapt explanation according to individual patient.

○ Explore prior knowledge (patient's medical history, family history, etc.).

○ Build on this knowledge if appropriate.

○ Use information gathered earlier about health belief and experiences.

○ Use clear and jargon-free language.

○ Explain any medical terms used.

○ Use diagrams and models.

○ Break information into chunks.

○ Write down important points if necessary.

○ Back up with leaflets, CD-ROMs, etc.

○ Ask patient to repeat important information.

○ Give patient frequent opportunities to ask for clarification.

○ Give patient time at the end of the explanation to ask questions.

○ Offer/arrange follow-up appointment for further discussion of queries.

Adapting the explanation to a patient's cognitive ability is highly skilful. It is easy to assume that patients from certain backgrounds do not assimilate information easily. It is easy to be patronising. Doctors have been shown to spend less time on explanation to patients of lower social class (as defined by their occupation).[4] Junior doctors in general practice pitch their explanations based on value judgements of patients' ability to understand. These value judgements are made by intuition and instinct as well as by knowing where the patient lives and assessing how the patient told their story.[5] Experienced GPs are likely to use such mechanisms, as well as having insight into their patients, which has often been built up over many consultations. But doctors have to be careful not to judge inaccurately, and should check out their assumptions.

Helping patients to help themselves

Patients with existing or recurrent problems, including diagnosed illnesses or symptoms for which a serious underlying cause has been excluded, should be encouraged to manage themselves. If information has been shared adequately between doctor and patient, and they have agreed on a management plan, the patient should not need to consult a doctor on every occasion of flare-up of symptoms; but regular review should be agreed as necessary.

Patient self-management is common in certain chronic diseases such as diabetes, asthma and arthritis. Specialist nurses advise patients of management strategies and encourage them to monitor their conditions, adjusting medication as appropriate. Patient education by doctors, nurses, pharmacists and the media helps patients to manage self-limiting illnesses such as colds and musculoskeletal pain.

The key to this approach is explanation. Doctors become teachers of their patients, but doctors also achieve a greater understanding of their patients' own experiences of illness. There is a learning experience on both sides.[6]

Negotiating and resolving conflict

○ **Negotiating** *to confer with another or others in order to come to terms or reach an agreement; to arrange or settle by discussion and mutual agreement.*

Step 6 in the shared decision-making process discussed in Chapter 3 is:

Make or negotiate a decision in partnership and resolve conflict.[7]

In the patient-centred approach the third component is finding common ground, which involves defining the problem, establishing the goals of treatment and identifying the roles to be assumed by doctor and patient.[8]

Many models of the processes involved in negotiation have been described in the literature of psychology, communication and business, but these are not particularly helpful in the medical scenario. Negotiation is not necessarily a process that doctors consider to be involved in consultations. Often patient and doctor will come to a mutual decision based on the information shared without any disagreement arising that needs settling.

However, in certain circumstances patient and doctor may have different ideas on which management option should be chosen. We have already seen that doctors may reduce potential conflict by only suggesting treatment options that they think are the best, the most cost effective or the most feasible in a given situation. If they do present a full range of options they have to be prepared that the patient may not choose one of the doctors' preferences. Patients also suggest treatments and these may have to be discussed. In the informed model the doctor leaves the patient to decide alone and no negotiation is required. In the shared model if there is disagreement, negotiation may be necessary.

How far should a doctor try to influence a patient's choice? It is easy to belittle certain options, particularly those that patients suggest. Oxfordshire GP and medical educator Peter Tate, in his influential text *The Doctor's Communication Handbook*, suggests that 'shepherding' techniques are useful influencing skills. He cites as an example how value-laden phrases can direct patients' choices. There is a difference between calling an osteopath 'a bloke that tweaks backs for £20 a time' or 'a colleague with more training in manipulation than me'.[9]

Consider also the situation in which the patient makes a decision that the doctor feels is detrimental to the patient's wellbeing, the family's or indeed society's as a whole. Concordance poses ethical and legal challenges in such scenarios.[10]

Common examples of potential conflicts are shown in Box 5.2. Some situations may involve more than one person. Some relate to patients having expectations that would fulfil their wants rather than their needs (see Chapter 3). However, we need to be careful, because the difference between wants and needs tends to be defined by doctors.

Box 5.2 ○ Examples of potential conflicts

○ Patient wanting antibiotics for a sore throat.

○ Parent not wishing child to have MMR vaccination.

○ Patient wishing to have an X-ray to screen for lung cancer.

○ Daughter wanting father to be admitted and father refuses.

○ Husband not wishing to disclose his HIV status to wife.

○ Patient unwilling to start treatment for TB.

○ Patient wishing to be referred for cardiac investigations when doctor believes chest pain is non-cardiac in origin.

○ Doctor wanting patient to be investigated for rectal bleeding and patient declining.

○ Patient wanting reversal of sterilisation.

○ Patient wanting home visit for back pain.

○ New patient wanting a prescription for strong painkillers or tranquillisers.

These conflicts arise even if the doctor has adopted a patient-centred approach, has explored the patient's ideas and concerns, explained the problem and possible diagnosis, and given a full description of options including evidence, advantages and disadvantages of each. Of course, in the real world such conflicts often arise because the doctor has not had time to do all this, the patient has not understood the explanation or the patient's previous experiences have left them unconvinced of the doctor's recommendations. Thus in certain circumstances conflict can be constructive, uncovering differences in values and legitimate concerns that have been inadequately discussed.[11] Doctor and patient may not have the same view of what will be a positive outcome from the consultation.

In the main doctors do not want to end consultations on a 'bad' note, with patients dissatisfied due to unmet needs or wants, and doctors feeling their knowledge and skills have been undervalued or undermined. In these conflict situations can doctor and patient find common ground and agree on a management plan, or indeed agree to disagree without harming the doctor–patient relationship?

Doctors may approach conflict situations believing that the patient is an adversary and that they need to 'win'. In these situations patients may be labelled as 'time wasters', 'malingerers' or manipulative. Or doctors may agree with the patient for the sake of speed and not wanting to upset the doctor–patient relationship. Both of these strategies have been criticised by Fisher and Ury, who suggest that a better way of negotiation is to focus on interests, not positions, and to try to be objective rather than simply pitting one personal opinion against another.[12] However, the medical consultation is dissimilar to negotiation in other circumstances. It is difficult to remain objective in the face of distress, sickness and/or aggression.

Ultimately the doctor has the power of the prescription pad and the referral letter, as the gatekeeper of the National Health Service within the UK. Patients have the power to decline a prescription or referral (as long as they are believed to be cognitively competent). Ethical questions arise in the grey area of private medicine. Are patients who are prepared to pay for certain investigations likely to be referred whereas other patients would not be referred?

There are no easy answers to these questions or simple ways of dealing with conflict scenarios, though empathic statements are very helpful (see pp. 84–5). All a doctor's skills are required but the doctor does need a willingness to accept the patient as an equal in terms of giving the patient time to express feelings. Ending a consultation feeling that you have 'given in' to a patient is destructive in the long run, but feeling that you have accepted the patient's viewpoint and negotiated the best-case scenario for both GP and patient is more rewarding. This may mean also taking into account the needs of the wider community. Doctors should decline certain patients' demands, but they also have to accept that patients will sometimes decline their recommendations.

Further issues regarding empathy

○ **Empathy** *identification with and understanding of another's situation, feelings and motives.*

○ **Empathy as defined by an educationalist** *'The ability to understand your own thoughts and feelings and, by analogy, apply your self-understanding to the service of others, mindful that their thinking and feeling might not match your own.'* [13]

'Empathy is the feeling that "I might be you" or "I am you", but is more than just an intellectual identification; empathy must be accompanied by feeling. Sympathy brings compassion, "I want to help you," but empathy brings emotion. Without feeling there is no empathy.' [14] A doctor may be sympathetic and understanding. A doctor may commiserate with a patient without placing or imagining himself or herself in the same position.

However, is empathy always a good thing in consultations? Criticism of the empathic doctor has been made on the grounds that such a doctor cannot act objectively and make the best decision. 'Encouraging physicians to cultivate empathy in their relations with patients will undermine their ability to function as wise, understanding doctors who give of themselves in guiding patients through life's concerns and illnesses.' [15] Perhaps the problem here is one of perception of the doctor's role. Does a GP expect to guide a patient in this way? Does good clinical decision making depend on the doctor being distant and unemotional? It is more likely that to be therapeutic doctors must connect with their patients on at least some emotional level to motivate them towards healing. [16]

However, doctors need to be careful of confusing what they would feel in a certain circumstance with what the patient is actually feeling. This tendency has been called 'pseudo-empathy'. [17] For example, the author Hilary Mantel in her memoir relates how she returned to see one GP after many years of misdiagnosis of her endometriosis. She was 27 at the time and informed the doctor of her female castration. The doctor replied 'There's one good thing, anyway. Now you won't have to worry about birth prevention.' [18] Perhaps this doctor assumed too much, that any woman would be glad of an end to such worry. On reflection we could probably all remember such inappropriate remarks made with the best intentions.

Empathy is a natural attribute that may be heightened by personal experience of illness or traumatic events, though even if a doctor has had a similar experience to a patient's, it will only be similar and not the same. Empathy may also be used as a technical skill to help develop rapport. After all, no doctor can experience every condition with which patients present. There-fore as a skill it may be learnt.[19] Empathy may be thought of as a two-stage process:

- the understanding and sensitive appreciation of another person's predica-ment or feelings

- the communication of the understanding back to the patient in a supportive way.[20]

There are both verbal and non-verbal components involved in demon-strating empathy. Non-verbal communication is used to show that the doc-tor is sensitive to the patient's feelings and may include lowering the voice, touching the patient's hand or being silent. Of course other skills are used, such as eye contact and listening. Verbal techniques centre on empathic statements and are used to link the 'I' of the doctor and the 'you' of the patient.[20] Examples relating to some of the conflict scenarios above are shown in Box 5.3.

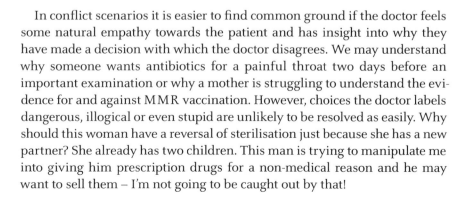

Box 5.3 ○ Empathic statements

○ I can see that you are in a lot of pain.

○ I can understand why you are worried about the MMR vaccination.

○ I can see that you are very worried about the possibility of lung cancer.

○ I realise how upsetting your father's condition is for you.

○ I appreciate how difficult if must be for you to tell your wife about this.

○ I can see that you are really worried about this pain because of your father's recent heart attack.

In conflict scenarios it is easier to find common ground if the doctor feels some natural empathy towards the patient and has insight into why they have made a decision with which the doctor disagrees. We may understand why someone wants antibiotics for a painful throat two days before an important examination or why a mother is struggling to understand the evi-dence for and against MMR vaccination. However, choices the doctor labels dangerous, illogical or even stupid are unlikely to be resolved as easily. Why should this woman have a reversal of sterilisation just because she has a new partner? She already has two children. This man is trying to manipulate me into giving him prescription drugs for a non-medical reason and he may want to sell them – I'm not going to be caught out by that!

Lack of empathy in certain situations is understandable. We cannot like all our patients, agree with all their decisions and not be affected by what we see as unreasonable demands. Doctors' own feelings and experiences will also limit empathy in some cases. John Salinsky and Paul Sackin, British GP course organisers working within a Balint framework of case discussion, have identified defensive overreactions in consultations that limit empathic responses. They suggest that certain warning signs should alert doctors who are putting up defences against emotional involvement (Box 5.4).[21]

Box 5.4 ○ Defensive strategies[21]

- ○ Anxiety.
- ○ Feeling irritable.
- ○ Worried about time.
- ○ Being withdrawn and aloof.
- ○ Being cold and contemptuous.
- ○ Anger.
- ○ Being careful not to offend.
- ○ Overuse of the biomedical model.
- ○ Apostolic behaviour.
- ○ Talking about health education.
- ○ Sticking firmly to practice policies.
- ○ Feeling too closely identified with the patient.

Doctors cannot function at the optimal level all the time. Recognition of such behaviour is important so that patient care is not compromised. At times like these perhaps it is best to be honest with the patient and say you cannot help at this moment. Ask the patient to make another appointment or see another doctor. You may wish to ask a colleague for advice or support, or simply discuss the case in order to sort out your own feelings.

Dealing with symptoms

○ **Symptom** *a sign or an indication of disorder or disease, especially when experienced by an individual as a change from normal function, sensation or appearance.*

Medical terminology describes patients as having presenting complaints. These are usually symptoms, e.g. headache, sore throat, back pain. Some people may give their symptoms a diagnosis dependent on their past experience, e.g. migraine, tonsillitis, slipped disc. In all these cases the doctors must explore the patient's story and find out exactly what the patient is experiencing.

Symptoms are common. Many people have symptoms without seeking medical help. One survey in the USA found that, of 1 million respondents, about half had a headache, a third fatigue and 15 per cent a sore throat at the moment they were asked about how they were feeling.[22] While these findings are 40 years old it is likely they are mirrored in people's experiences today. Doctors may be thankful that only a small proportion of these people seek medical help, suggesting that most people do not regard their symptoms as being illnesses or warranting medical intervention.[23]

Of those patients who do visit a GP, most will have minor illnesses or conditions, some will have serious illnesses and many will remain as 'medically unexplained'. In another US study of 1000 consultations involving patients with 14 different common acute symptoms, doctors diagnosed an organic illness in 16 per cent, a psychological problem in 10 per cent and in the remaining 74 per cent the cause of the symptoms remained unknown.[24] Of course, following up the patients may have revealed further pathological diagnoses, though many of the symptoms would probably be self-limiting. However, the three types of scenario are challenging in different ways. The main strategy for each is for the doctor to elicit the patient's story and adopt a patient-centred approach, as has already been described in detail.

Leaving symptoms unexplained is frustrating and dissatisfying for both patient[25] and doctor.[26] One or both may be concerned that serious pathology is being overlooked. This concern should be brought into the open. The doctor may ask specifically 'Are you afraid it is something serious?' Or be more indirect: 'Are you worried about something?' The doctor may be able to explain the symptoms within a medical framework and indeed this may help the patient. Recent advances in our understanding of irritable bowel syndrome (IBS), for example, suggest that both central and peripheral neural components are important in the pathogenesis of IBS, resulting in the development of the concept of the brain–gut axis[27] that may be affected by stress. However, it is tempting to suggest medical reasons for symptoms without being sure of any underlying causes. From there it is common to prescribe for the symptoms without tackling any such underlying cause. Uncertainty regarding diagnosis is one factor that influences doctors to prescribe.[28] However, if the symptoms do not resolve, the patient is likely to reappear and another prescription is given or investigations are ordered.

Some of the patients dealt with in this manner may go on to become frequent attenders or be labelled as heartsink patients. However, some of them may eventually be diagnosed with 'real' pathology. For 10 years Hilary Mantel's symptoms were diagnosed as psychosomatic, then as depression, until finally she was found to have extensive endometriosis.[18]

So what can be done in these consultations? Doctor and patient need to live with the uncertainty. The patient-centred framework and shared decision making with good communication skills should help alleviate the burden. Follow-up is essential if issues are unresolved. Listening and reassessment are important.

'Heartsink' patients and frequent attenders

This group of patients is a challenge in general practice. O'Dowd, previously a GP in Nottingham and now professor in Dublin, coined the term 'heartsink' in 1988.[29] Ten years earlier, showing how times have changed, a US psychiatrist called Groves talked of 'hateful' patients.[30] Not all heartsink patients are frequent attenders but many frequent attenders cause the heart to sink, often because doctors want to help and they are unable to do so in certain situations. Research findings and strategies to help these patients are often published together in the general practice literature. Groves's classification (Box 5.5) is of historical interest, presenting as it does an image of

---

Box 5.5 ○ Groves's 1978 classification of 'hateful' patients[30]

○ **The dependent clinger** • excessively dependent of the doctor. Desperate for reassurance. Returns frequently with new symptoms, but is grateful for the doctor's attention.

○ **The entitled demander** • intimidates, devalues and induces guilt. Demands referrals if expectations not met.

○ **The manipulative help-rejecter** • nothing ever works. Often sees other doctors.

○ **The self-destructive denier** • cannot accept that own bad habits are causing symptoms and will make no significant alterations in lifestyle.

---

the medical profession that saw fit to use non-patient-centred definitions. GPs can all recognise some of their own patients in these descriptions, but would hesitate (hopefully) to use such pejorative terms. Classifications like this are useful in deflecting emotions and in de-stressing with colleagues but are not really helpful in tackling the underlying problems. In many ways they reflect a failure on the part of the doctor to explore a patient's problems and may be used as an excuse not to engage fully with a patient's needs. Frequent attenders are in fact a quite heterogeneous group of patients, with a variety of needs including genuine health care, but with the common characteristic of consulting at least once every month.[31] It is chastening to think that for some patients the only meaningful conversation they have is with a health professional. The surgery is a point of social contact for the isolated and lonely people without family support.

The label 'medically unexplained symptoms'[32] is thought to be scientifically neutral. However, one study has shown that patients prefer the word 'functional', in its original sense of altered functioning of the nervous system, to what they perceive as a non-diagnosis of medically unexplained.[33] One group of patients has been defined as having chronic multiple functional somatic symptoms (CMFS), a term that is being used in preference to somatisation disorder.[34] About 4 per cent of the general population has CMFS, most of them women: an average of 10–15 per GP.[34] Other features of these patients are: age over 40; living alone; multiple referrals for physical symptoms; having fear of organic cause, often cancer; depression and/or anxiety; family problems; and lack of insight.

Dealing with these types of patients engenders many different emotions in the doctor. Empathy is often lost, while anger and frustration are common. Doctors despair of ever being able to help or resolve the patients' problems. They wonder why these patients keep coming back to see them. The doctor may verbalise this frustration: 'You have been coming to see me for a while now and I don't really feel that I have helped you. What do you think we should do now?' Or empathise with the patient's own presumed frustration: 'The fact that I haven't been able to help you must be very frustrating.'

When GPs first encounter patients like this they do not label them immediately. There are few warning signs. Even the old 'fat folder' sign has disappeared due to computerisation. It is often only when the frequent attendance has become a pattern and the doctor recognises the signs of frustration that a 'diagnosis' is made. Going back to basics and using all the communication skills at one's disposal are important strategies in management. A full history including the patient-centred approach is helpful in enabling both doctor and patient to share information. Certain life events may come to light that the patient has never volunteered previously. Or these may have been lost in the mountain of paperwork and hospital letters. Discovering the patient's story may restore the doctor's empathy and, though it may not offer management solutions immediately, such knowledge should improve the doctor–patient relationship.

A framework for consultations with frequent attenders and 'difficult' patients is shown in Box 5.6. Some of this has been adapted from Bass and May's work on CMFS.[34] Not all these steps can or should be covered in one consultation. It is important to remember that it is the doctor-centred professional who labels patients as 'difficult'. It is likely that patients have similar feelings about some doctors. 'Difficult' in this context means that a doctor is unable to formulate a diagnosis and management plan because of a failure on the doctor's part to elicit the patient's story or consider any problems outside a strict biomedical model.

However, once a patient's story has been elicited, doctors must be careful not to attempt to 'psychoanalyse' the patient. It is easy to conjecture that a patient's symptoms relate to a particular life event. This may be the case and the patient may also see links between event and illness. However, the two may not be cause and effect. We may hope that making such links will resolve some of the patient's problems and then both patient and doctor are disappointed when this does not happen. Life is usually more complicated than it may at first appear. Do not be tempted to reduce a patient's probably multifactorial condition to a simple model. The process is similar to being directive when counselling.

Listing these steps makes the process seem easy, but of course it is not. GPs need support with these difficult consultations, which could be discussed at clinical practice meetings or local support groups.

Patients with 'symptoms' and frequent attenders ○ *reflections*

As a junior doctor I wasn't really taught how to manage patients without 'real' illnesses. General practice was a shock. The familiar patterns of ward-based disease were missing. Patients might have one single symptom that made no sense or a combination of symptoms and signs that suggested multiple and illogical pathology. I learnt how to unravel these problems with experience and time, watching how certain symptoms resolved and how some were related to life changes and other external factors. But there is always that frisson of uncertainty. Just as the patient is concerned that the doctor is missing a vital diagnosis, so am I. Once you know about a patient with bowel cancer at 28 and breast cancer even younger, you become more wary of suggesting alternative, usually stress-related, diagnoses. One of my patients in her late forties, whose youngest daughter aged 15 concealed her pregnancy until 24 weeks' gestation, started to experience bloating and abdominal discomfort as her daughter neared delivery. Examination was normal. But eventually she was diagnosed as having ovarian cancer.

Box 5.6 ○ Stages in the process of dealing with 'difficult' patients

Prior to the consultation: review the patient's records including investigations, referrals and treatments with their timeframe. Information gathering:

○ gather information about the presenting complaint

○ elicit the patient's story including social background and life events

○ use open questions and try not to adopt a biomedical model

○ gather information about the previous medical history and its timeframe in the patient's own words, including treatment and the patient's feeling about this

○ explore the patient's ideas, concerns and expectations

○ do not assume that the patient wants investigations or a prescription (see Chapter 3)

○ discuss the patient's experiences with medical services and previous doctors, and find out why they have consulted you today

○ reframe the physical symptoms if possible to show links between life events (with caution)

○ remember to reflect on how you are feeling as this may mirror the patient's mood, e.g. frustrated, angry

○ it may be relevant and appropriate to ask a family member or friend to see you with the patient at a later stage.

Information sharing, shared decision making and management:

○ formulate a problem list with the patient and priorities for management

○ discuss the probability that there is no cure but rather an improvement in wellbeing to some extent and that this will take time

○ discuss the use of any drugs, prescribed or OTC (over the counter), and decide which are necessary

○ check that the patient has understood

○ encourage patient to take responsibility for health

○ avoid referral

○ make informal contract with patient to consult with you only and at predefined intervals

○ involve family member or friend to help support patient in managing the problems.

Patients with disabilities

Communication difficulties arise with patients with a variety of disabilities including stroke, cerebral palsy, deafness and Parkinson's disease. While each situation is different, there are generic skills that may be used to overcome problems. The doctor may have difficulty understanding the patient due to speech and articulation impediments. The patient may have difficulty understanding the doctor because of hearing impairment or limited language skills. The doctor needs to assess the level and nature of the patient's disability, bearing in mind that not all patients with communication problems have intellectual impairment. This is important, as the doctor should try to interact directly with the patient when at all possible.

Often the patient will come to the surgery with a carer or relative. This person should be able to give information about the patient's communication needs and strategies for dealing with them appropriately. Patients may not be able to verbalise their problems and needs, but other methods are available, such as body language – including facial expressions and gestures – signing, communication boards and books, and electronic systems.

Some strategies for aiding communication are shown in Box 5.7.[35]

Box 5.7 ○ **Communication strategies for patients with disabilities**[35]
○ Direct questions to and discussion with the patient when possible.
○ Recommend a double consultation as required.
○ Do not worry about silences – patients may need time to process information.
○ Do not talk while the patient is considering a reply.
○ Repeat the patient's answers as appropriate to ensure that you have understood.
○ Find out if the patient has specific signs for certain common words such as yes and no.
○ Use the same signs if possible.
○ Ask permission before involving the carer or relative.

Breaking bad news

Bad news comes in many forms, though breaking it is often thought of only when giving a diagnosis of cancer. Robert Buckman, a British oncologist now working in Toronto, has defined bad or unfavourable news as 'any news that drastically and negatively alters the patient's view of her or his future'.[36] How can a doctor know how a patient's view will be altered?

When confirming a patient's pregnancy the astute doctor will not assume that the result is welcomed. It is easy to assume that our perception of bad news is exactly the same as that of our patients. Within the paternalistic framework of medical practice, doctors tried to shield their patients from poor prognoses, even considering it inhumane or detrimental to patients to be honest about diagnoses.[37] The patient-centred approach and shared decision-making model encourage doctors to be more open in information sharing and management planning. This openness and honesty is in line with the wishes of patients who have been shown to want to know if their diagnosis is cancer.[38] Moreover, how bad news is broached affects patients' psychological adjustment,[39] demonstrating the importance of the doctors' skills in this difficult area.

Breaking bad news should never be considered in isolation. All the consultation skills described and considered so far, the slow building of a doctor–patient relationship, the establishment of rapport and the sharing of information prepare both doctor and patient for difficult interviews in the future. If doctor and patient know each other, the task, while daunting, should be less difficult. Moreover, when a good doctor–patient relationship exists already, the doctor should be less likely to try to avoid giving a diagnosis and discussing management.

So the groundwork for this task begins when, or even before, a patient presents with symptoms that are potentially serious. When the doctor explores the patient's ideas and concerns, the patient's anxiety regarding a possible diagnosis such as cancer is elicited. The doctor may be able to gauge how the patient will react to the possibility becoming reality and have some idea of what and how the patient would like to be told. A difficult dilemma is how much to prepare a patient when history and examination strongly suggest malignancy, but the doctor is not completely certain of the diagnosis until all the investigations are complete. How much do you tell the patient? False reassurance is not appropriate. Honesty at this stage is helpful later, and certainly a patient's questions should be answered truthfully. Trust is important and betrayal of this trust will harm the therapeutic relationship. But each case is different and some of the truth could be withheld until later; the patient should only be told what they want to know.

Once the diagnosis is certain it will not always be the GP who breaks the news, but the GP will certainly be involved in care. The GP may need to help a patient for whom the news was not broken in quite the best way. When following up patients after hospital visits it is important to find out what the patient has been told. In the scenario where the GP has to give a bad result following open-access investigations, the news should be given in small chunks, checking that the patient understands as the story unfolds.

Doctors will develop their own personal ways of showing sensitivity and of course empathy. A box of tissues on the desk, ample time and preparation are important. It is not good practice to look for a result while the patient is waiting in the consulting room. There is no time to think about what to say and to think about how the patient may react.

Baile, Buckman and colleagues have developed a six-step protocol for breaking bad news, which they have called SPIKES (Box 5.8).[40] While part of step 6 is concerned with treatment options and is more applicable to be carried out by a specialist, the framework is useful for all doctors, especially as bad news may not only be related to malignancy. For example a GP may also have to give patients results of HIV and antenatal screening tests.

Gauging how much information the patient wants is a difficult part of the process. By asking questions about the patient's perceptions of what is happening, it may become apparent that bad news needs to be confirmed rather than broken.[41] If the patient appears to have no idea that the news is going to be bad the doctor may ask a question such as: 'Do you know what this test was for?' A signposting statement may be made: 'I'm afraid that the news isn't as good as we hoped.'[20] There is no one way to do this and much depends on what was said in the prior consultation when tests were ordered and the patient's concerns explored. This shows the importance of continuity of care.

Approach with caution the desire to give a prognosis. If such a step is vital, the most appropriate person to do this is the specialist, as treatments change and survival rates alter. Certainly be sure that all health professionals involved in the case are saying the same thing. Patients have a need for information about prognosis and how likely this is to be accurate. They feel it is important to be able to refine their understanding about prognosis as the disease progresses. However, they also want the provision of hope and express a need for hopeful messages at all stages.[42]

Denial by the patient is common and the bad news may need to be broken more than once. The patient ultimately has the right to know and pressure from relatives not to give the full diagnosis should be avoided. Relatives indeed should not really be informed about the medical condition before the patient, except in special circumstances. If relatives do ask for the patient not to be told, the reasons for this need to be explored. The doctor needs to remember that such collusion is because the relatives love the patient and want to spare them from extra distress.

It is important not to forget patients' perspective of how bad news should be broken, and the need to adapt the protocol for each individual. Patients value not only the doctors' interpersonal and communication skills, but also their technical competence and up-to-date knowledge.[43] Patients have

Box 5.8 ○ SPIKES protocol[40]

Step 1 ● SETTING up the interview

○ Arrange privacy and make sure there will be no interruptions.

○ Involve significant others as appropriate.

○ Sit down.

○ Connect with the patient: eye contact, touch.

○ Advise the patient of the time you have available.

Step 2 ● assessing the patient's PERCEPTION

○ Use open-ended questions: 'What have you been told about your condition so far?'

○ Gather information to explore the patient's perception of the situation.

○ Explore ideas, concerns and expectations.

○ Correct misinformation as necessary.

○ Helps determine whether the patient is in denial.

Step 3 ● obtaining the patient's INVITATION

○ Find out how the patient would like to receive the information (this is a useful step at the time of ordering tests, so both doctor and patient are prepared for the way the results should be given).

○ Gauge how much information the patient wants.

Step 4 ● giving KNOWLEDGE and information to the patient

○ Warn the patient that bad news is coming: 'Unfortunately I've got some bad news to tell you.'

○ Break information into small chunks.

○ Use appropriate language and check for understanding of each chunk of information.

Step 5 ● addressing the patient's EMOTIONS with empathic responses

○ Look out for the patient's emotional reaction.

○ Identify the emotion, e.g. anger, sadness.

○ Identify the reason for the emotion, asking the patient if necessary.

○ Make an empathic statement to acknowledge the emotion.

Step 6 ● STRATEGY and SUMMARY

○ Present treatment options.

○ Shared decision making.

○ Reach consensus.

○ Plan follow-up.

identified six attributes as important in doctors' communication of information when the bad news is first conveyed: playing it straight (being honest and direct); staying the course (not abandoning patients later in the illness); giving time; showing they care (empathy and compassion); making it clear (avoiding jargon); and pacing information.[42] However, doctors need to consider the patient's gender, age and educational background when deciding how much information to give, as it appears that women and patients with more formal education want more information.[44]

Motivational interviewing

This is another useful consultation technique that was initially introduced in the 1980s and refined by Miller and Rollnick in 1991.[45] It is based on the five stages of change model (Box 5.9).[46]

> ### Box 5.9 ○ Five stages of change model
>
> ① **Precontemplation** • patient has no intention to change behaviour in the foreseeable future. The patient is perhaps unaware that there is a problem.
>
> ② **Contemplation** • patient aware that problem exists and is thinking about changing behaviour but has no firm commitment to take action.
>
> ③ **Preparation** • patient intends to change in the next month.
>
> ④ **Action** • patient begins to modify behaviour to overcome the problem. This requires considerable commitment and energy.
>
> ⑤ **Maintenance and relapse prevention** • patient works to prevent relapse. This stage may last for many months or years.

Motivational interviewing is built upon the premise that if a person's idea of change were entirely positive, then altering behaviour would be easy. As with other consultation techniques, it is important in this approach to develop a safe and supportive rapport with the patient. The goals of motivational interviewing are listed in Box 5.10. Skills for motivational interviewing are no different from those we use in other circumstances to improve consultation outcomes. Listening, summarising and supporting are important. Double-sided reflection is helpful, i.e. 'So on the one hand you find that drinking alcohol initially makes you feel happy and less stressed, but on the other hand you know it makes you feel more aggressive and then ill the next day.'

Once the doctor has decided that a patient's behaviour is putting their health at risk, the doctor needs to identify which stage they are at in order to intervene in the most appropriate manner. In stage 1 the doctor's role is to engage patients in contemplating change. During this stage, patients may appear argumentative, hopeless or in 'denial', and the natural tendency is for doctors to try to 'convince' them, which usually engenders resistance.[47]

Patients may stay in stage 2 for many years and doctor and patient should explore the barriers to change. In stage 3 patients require information and support. During the maintenance stage, follow-up and further support is necessary. This support may be provided by other members of the primary healthcare team.

Box 5.10 ○ Goals of motivational interviewing

- ○ To help the patient explore their own behaviour.
- ○ To explore the advantages and disadvantages of a change in behaviour.
- ○ To look at how to overcome potential resistance to change.
- ○ To facilitate the patient's readiness for change.
- ○ To empower the patient to take responsibility for own health.
- ○ To set goals.
- ○ To help the patient develop realistic ways of changing behaviour.
- ○ To create a safe environment for the discussion.
- ○ To improve the patient's self-esteem.

Dealing with aggression

Patients become angry in consultations when conflict arises and their wants or demands are unmet, when they receive adverse news or during emotional and stressful interviews. Anger is common but aggression is rare. Patients with a history of violence or substance abuse are more likely to switch to aggression, and this may occur in patients of any age.[48] Doctors need to be able to deal with these situations. The anger and aggression may be directed at the doctor, though often receptionists or other healthcare staff receive the brunt of the patient's dissatisfaction. For those rarer cases where doctors or other staff feel or are physically intimidated or threatened by patients, a panic button should be available in surgery rooms.

Signs that a person is becoming angry include an increase in respiratory rate, speech becoming louder, facial flushing and obvious tension in the neck and shoulder. If a patient becomes angry it is important to acknowledge this and to explore the reasons for the emotion while not invading the patient's personal space. Empathic statements are helpful such as 'I can see that you are angry.' Simple statements of fact followed by invitations to discuss the problem may be made such as 'I noticed that you were very angry with the receptionist. Would you like to tell me why?' When dealing with an angry or confrontational patient there are certain strategies that can be employed (Box 5.11). Staff need to be supported but yourself becoming angry at the patient is usually more destructive for both doctor and patient. It is helpful to apologise to patients if they have been kept waiting past their appointment time. In fact anger may be defused if the receptionist keeps the patients informed of any delays and the reasons for them. It is not knowing what is happening that often makes patients anxious and subsequently angry. Conflicts that are discussed in private, at the right speed and time, without time pressures and with prior thought if possible, are more likely to be resolved with mutual satisfaction.[49]

Box 5.11 ○ Strategies for dealing with angry patients

○ Do not stand up to confront an angry person: invite the person to sit down.

○ If both of you are standing up, sit down yourself and then invite the person to sit down.

○ Move to a private room if appropriate, ensuring that your personal safety is not compromised.

○ Offer the person an appointment to come back and discuss the matter if you cannot sort out the problem immediately.

○ Use an appropriate tone of voice: do not shout or speak over the person.

○ Squarely face the other person and maintain eye contact.

○ Appear confident and professional.

○ Do not hunch or squirm.

○ Be firm as appropriate.

○ Do not give in to rash demands.

○ Allow time to de-stress after the interview: do not rush back into seeing patients.

We all make mistakes in diagnosis and treatment. These days it is accepted practice to apologise for any mistakes and to explain to the patient what has happened. This is a very difficult thing to do but may restore the patient's (and family's) lost faith and also deflect a complaint. Being honest is usually the best way to proceed. However, it is important to ensure that you are safe and that violence cannot escalate. Doctors should ensure they do not put themselves in vulnerable situations.

NLP

NLP was developed in the 1970s in California by a mathematician, Richard Bandler, and a linguistics professor, John Grinder. They wanted to understand how successful people achieve their success and then use this understanding to help other people excel. They defined NLP as the study of the structure of subjective experience and what can be calculated from that.[50] Their methods have been put into practice by psychologists and therapists, and more lately by doctors including general practitioners.

There are three parts to NLP (Box 5.12).[51] It is a useful and different way to look at consultation skills, but comes with its own jargon, much of which can be translated into more familiar words concerned with doctor–patient interactions. Further consideration is outside the scope of this book.

Box 5.12 ○ The three parts of NLP

Neuro • how we use out neurology to think and feel.

Linguistic • how we use language to influence others and ourselves.

Programming • how we act to achieve the goals that we set.

Dealing with aggression ○ *reflections*

I was thumped in the face by a drunken women in casualty while working there as an SHO (senior house officer, three years post-qualification). I was on my own with her. I didn't see such patients alone again. Luckily as a GP I have not been confronted with physical violence though I have been sworn at and shouted at on several occasions. Patients also threaten in more subtle ways – 'I'll report you if you don't do what I want.' Some patients are more likely to try manipulation or to lie. Doctors are vulnerable; not all patients are saints and frail. The best learning experience I had was working through a scenario with a simulated patient who was trying to obtain extra benzodiazepines. The scenario involved the reception staff and the pharmacist. I was shaking at the end, even though I had worked with the patient before. In the feedback session we were able to work through different methods of dealing with aggression, and felt more confident. The shift in the on-call system so that more GPs travel in cars with drivers is a good move. Single doctors are vulnerable to attack and we really should not be put into such positions these days. It is sad that sometimes we distrust our patients, or their families, or their environment, but this is a fact of modern life.

Difficult patients, difficult doctors ○ *reflections*

Like many friends and colleagues (including GPs when they were patients or carers), I've done my share of working out how to deal with my 'difficult doctor'. I guess we too try to think of things from their perspective. Sometimes we manipulate, like hiding our medical, insider knowledge, in case we don't get straightforward advice or it gets our doctor's back up. I remember working with a group of women from a large housing estate. They were trying, and failing, to get across to their doctors what they felt they needed. There was a lot of 'empathy work' going on – 'They're so busy', 'I suppose he thinks this or that', 'I do wonder how they cope', etc. They tried 'the dreaded role-play' too. In the end, they practised asserting their thoughts clearly and kindly – or taking a mate with them who could do it for them. It seemed to work. We don't know what their doctors thought – but I like to think they appreciated it. Who wants to carry on in a fog of misunderstanding? It's all about how to get through to someone more powerful than you. It's a shame when our fear, as patient or doctor, gets in the way of empathy.

○ Summary

- Doctors may find it helpful to give details to patients in the three domains of explaining: interpretive; descriptive; and reason giving.

- The doctor must consider the existing knowledge and beliefs of the patient.

- A patient's lack of understanding may not be apparent until decisions about treatment are necessary.

- Some conflict situations relate to patients having expectations that would fulfil their wants rather than their needs.

- In certain circumstances conflict can be constructive, uncovering differences in a patient's values and legitimate concerns that have been inadequately discussed.

- Doctor and patient may not have the same view of what will be a positive outcome from the consultation.

- Doctors should decline certain patients' demands, but they also have to accept that patients will sometimes decline their recommendations.

- There are both verbal and non-verbal components involved in demonstrating empathy.

- Empathy is an attribute but it may also be used as a technical skill to help develop rapport.

- Leaving symptoms unexplained is frustrating and dissatisfying for both patient and doctor.

- The patient ultimately has the right to know 'bad news' and pressure from relatives not to give the full diagnosis should be avoided.

REFERENCES

1 Katz R L. *Empathy: Its Nature and Uses*. New York: Free Press, 1963.

2 Brown G and Atkins M. Explaining. In: Hargie O D W (ed.). *The Handbook of Communication Skills*. Second edition. London: Routledge, 1997, pp. 183–212.

3 Ausubel D P, Novak J S and Hanesian H. *Educational Psychology: A Cognitive View*. Second edition. New York: Rinehart & Wilson, 1978.

4 Pendleton D and Bochner S. The communication of medical information in general practice consultations as a function of social class. *Social Science and Medicine* 1980; **14**: 669–73.

5 Thistlethwaite J E and van der Vleuten C. Informed shared decision making: views and competencies of pre-registration house officers in hospital and general practice. *Education for Primary Care* 2004; **15**: 83–92.

6 Herxheimer A. Helping patients take responsibility for their own health. *Annals of Internal Medicine* 2001; **135**: 51–2.

7 Towle A, Godolphin W and Richardson A. *Competencies for Informed Shared Decision-Making (ISDM): Report on Interviews with Physicians, Patients and Patient Educators and Focus Group Meetings with Patients*. Vancouver: University of British Columbia, 1997.

8 Stewart M, Brown J B, Weston W W, McWhinney I R, McWilliam C L and Freeman T R. *Patient-Centered Medicine. Transforming the Clinical Method*. California: Sage, 1995.

9 Tate P. *The Doctor's Communication Handbook*. Abingdon: Radcliffe Medical Press, 1994, p. 70.

10 Jones G. Prescribing and taking medicines. *BMJ* 2003; **327**: 819.

11 Way J, Back A L and Curtis J R. Withdrawing life support and resolution of conflict with families. *BMJ* 2002; **325**: 1342–5.

12 Fisher R and Ury W. *Getting to Yes: Negotiating Agreement without Giving in*. New York: Penguin, 1983.

13 Arnold R. *Empathic Intelligence. Teaching, Learning, Relating.* Sydney: UNSW Press, 2005, p. 23.

14 Spiro HM. Empathy: an introduction. In: Spiro H, Curnen MGM, Peschel E and St James D (eds). *Empathy and the Practice of Medicine.* New Haven: Yale University Press, 1993, pp. 1–6.

15 Landau RL. ... And the least of these is empathy. In: Spiro H, Curnen MGM, Peschel E and St James D (eds). *Empathy and the Practice of Medicine.* New Haven: Yale University Press, 1993, pp. 103–9.

16 Coulehan JL. Tenderness and steadiness: emotions in medical practice. *Literature and Medicine* 1995; **14**: 222–36.

17 Rosenfield PJ and Jones L. Striking a balance: training medical students to provide empathic care. *Medical Education* 2004; **38**: 927–33.

18 Mantel H. *Giving up the Ghost. A Memoir.* London: Harper Perennial, 2004, p. 211.

19 Platt VW and Keller VF. Empathic communication: a teachable and learnable skill. *Journal of General Internal Medicine* 1994; **9**: 222–6.

20 Silverman J, Kurtz S and Draper J. *Skills for Communicating with Patients.* Abingdon: Radcliffe Medical Press, 1998, pp. 83–4.

21 Salinsky J and Sackin P. *What Are You Feeling Doctor? Identifying and Avoiding Defensive Patterns in the Consultation.* Abingdon: Radcliffe Medical Press, 2000, p. 133.

22 Hammond EC. Some preliminary findings on physical complaints from a prospective study of 1,064,004 men and women. *American Journal of Public Health* 1964; **54**: 11–23.

23 Komaroff AL. Symptoms: in the head or in the brain? *Annals of Internal Medicine* 2001; **134**: 783–5.

24 Kroenke K and Mangelsdorff AD. Common symptoms in ambulatory care: incidence, evaluation, therapy and outcome. *American Journal of Medicine* 1989; **86**: 262–6.

25 Jackson AL and Kroenke K. The effect of unmet expectations among adults presenting with physical symptoms. *Annals of Internal Medicine* 2001; **134**: 889–97.

26 Hahn SR. Physical symptoms and physician-experienced difficulty in the physician–patient relationship. *Annals of Internal Medicine* 2001; **134**: 897–904.

27 Bose M and Farthing MJG. Irritable bowel syndrome: new horizons in pathophysiology and treatment. *British Journal of Surgery* 2001; **88**: 1425–6.

28 Bradley CP. Factors which influence the decision whether or not to prescribe: the dilemma facing general practitioners. *BJGP* 1992; **42**: 454–8.

29 O'Dowd TC. Five years of heartsink patients in general practice. *BMJ* 2002; **325**: 1342–5.

30 Groves JE. Taking care of the hateful patient. *New England Journal of Medicine* 1978; **298**: 317–18.

31 Neal R. Frequent attenders: who needs treatment? *BJGP* 1996; **46**: 131–2.

32 Reid S, Wessely S, Crayford T and Hotopf M. Medically unexplained symptoms in frequent attenders of secondary health care: retrospective cohort study. *BMJ* 2001; **322**: 767–71.

33 Stone J, Wojcik W, Durrance D, *et al.* What should we say to patients with symptoms unexplained by disease? The 'number needed to offend'. *BMJ* 2002; **325**: 1449–50.

34 Bass C and May S. Chronic multiple functional somatic symptoms. *BMJ* 2002; **325**: 323–6.

35 Iacono T and Johnson H. Patients with disabilities and complex communication needs. The GP consultation. *Australian Family Physician* 2004; **33**: 585–9.

36 Buckman R. *How to Break Bad News: A Guide for Health Professionals.* Baltimore: Johns Hopkins Press, 1992.

37 Oken D. What to tell cancer patients: a study of medical attitudes. *Journal of the American Medical Association* 1961; **175**: 1120–8.

38 Meredith C, Symonds P, Webster L, *et al.* Information needs of cancer patients in west Scotland: cross sectional survey of patients' views. *BMJ* 1996; **313**: 724–6.

39 Roberts C S, Cox C E, Reintgen D S, *et al.* Influence of physician communication on newly diagnosed patients' psychologic adjustment and decision making. *Cancer* 1994; **74**: 336–41.

40 Baile W F, Buckman R, Lenzi R, *et al.* SPIKES – a six-step protocol for delivering bad news: application to the patient with cancer. *The Oncologist* 2000; **5**: 302–11.

41 Faulkner A. ABC of palliative care: communication with patients, families and other professionals. *BMJ* 1998; **316**: 130–2.

42 Kirk P, Kirk I and Kristjanson C J. What do patients receiving palliative care for cancer and their families want to be told? An Australian and Canadian qualitative study. *BMJ* 2004; **328**: 1343, doi:10.1136/bmj.38103.423576.55.

43 Wiggers J H, Donovan K O, Redman S, *et al.* Cancer patients' satisfaction with care. *Cancer* 1990; **66**: 610–16.

44 Parker P A, Baile W F, de Moor C, *et al.* Breaking bad news about cancer: patients' preferences for communication. *Journal of Clinical Oncology* 2001; **19**: 2049–56.

45 Miller W and Rollnick S. *Motivational Interviewing: Preparing People to Change Addictive Behaviour.* New York: Guilford Press, 1991.

46 Prochaska J O, DiClemente C C and Norcross J C. In search of how people change. *American Psychologist* 1992; **47**: 1102–4.

47 Zimmerman G L, Olsen C G and Bosworth M F. A 'stages of change' approach to helping patients change behaviour. *American Family Physician* 2000; **61**: 1409–16.

48 Cembrowicz S, Rutter S and Wright S. Attacks on doctors and nurses. In: Shepherd J (ed.). *Violence in Healthcare.* Second edition. Oxford: Oxford University Press, 2001.

49 Rakos R F. Asserting and confronting. In: Hargie O D W (ed.) *The Handbook of Communication Skills.* Second edition. London: Routledge, 1997, pp. 289–319.

50 Bandler R and Grinder J. *Frogs into Princes.* Utah: Real People Press, 1979.

51 Walker L. *Consulting with NLP. Neuro-linguistic Programming in the Medical Consultation.* Oxford: Radcliffe Medical Press, 2002.

Issues relating to changes in general practice affecting the doctor–patient relationship

This chapter explores:

- the changing role of general practitioners due to changes in society ● the effects of consultation length ● issues relating to continuity of care ● quality of care and consultation factors ● the concept of cultural competency ● racism within medicine ● working with interpreters and patient advocates ● issues relating to refugee patients ● the GP and social justice ● the educational role of the GP.

'General practitioners are a bunch of individualists, perhaps the last professional generalists, impossible to deal with as a group but useful to have around when you need them. It cannot be overemphasized how profoundly the growth of central control and management technology threatens their traditional role. For a traditional role it is – there is an ecological niche for something of the kind in virtually all societies and at every point in history. But now the clash of cultures appears to be irreconcilable.'

JAMES WILLIS[1]

Society and medicine are changing all the time. We have explored the evolution of the doctor–patient relationship within the consultation from one of inequality and paternalism to one of patient partnership and shared decision making. This development is taking place at a time when British society is very different from that of even 20 years ago. On the whole people are better informed through greater access to the media, including the internet, and are more likely to challenge the opinions of professionals, while also showing less deference than previously to figures of authority. Medical undergraduate training is hopefully preparing the doctors of tomorrow to interact with this changing population of patients. Practising doctors must also realise that general practice is not what it was and adapt their skills to meet the needs of varying sets of patients, including patients from different cultures and with different customs.

We may lament the changes to the profession. However, not all these developments are externally driven. Many general practitioners are no longer prepared to work the long hours of their predecessors. In the UK the 24-hour responsibility for patient care has been removed from the individual doctor.

Changes in the general practitioner's role, general practice itself and patient profile are shown in Table 6.1.

Table 6.1 ○ **Changes affecting general practice and GPs**

General practice	Role of and demands on GP	Patient profile
Smaller list sizes	Emphasis on health promotion	Ageing
Larger partnerships	Emphasis on disease prevention	Multicultural
Fewer home visits	Member of team	Social deprivation
Special clinics	Specialist interests	Smaller families
Loss of personal lists	Often part time	Consumerism
Loss of continuity of care	More female doctors	Mobile
Longer consultations	Less likely to work out of hours	Litigious
Pressure to reduce prescribing	Financial awareness	Going private
Pressure to cut costs	Lifelong learning	High demand
Pressure to improve quality	Revalidation	Internet access
Appraisal	Guidelines	Walk-in centres
Protocols	Education of medical students	Loss of deference to authority figures

Research into the consultation

The consultation, its length, quality and communication, patient satisfaction and outcomes, are all big business in the research community. Slowly some research findings filter down into everyday practice. Many are lost amongst the pages of print that GPs try to assimilate each week. While most GPs try to keep up-to-date with advances in medical science and therapeutics as applied to them and their patients, the literature of general practice process and development is perhaps not so pressing. Such reading may be necessary for membership examinations and for the aspiring GP trainer, but is of low priority for many harassed doctors trying to get to grips with the latest guidelines and antihypertensive treatments. Just as GPs may ask 'What implications does this have for my patients?' of evidence-based data, they may also ask 'What implications does this paper on doctor–patient communication have for me?' Often, sadly, very few.

Ask yourself: if I don't read the *British Medical Journal* every week, or the *British Journal of General Practice* every month, what harm will befall me or my patients? However, the fact that you are reading this book shows you have an interest in communication and the consultation.

This chapter will not digest and make sense of as much published evidence as the others. But rather it will offer a view of the consultation within the early years of the 21st century and ask whether GPs need to change the way they practise in relation to doctor–patient interaction in everyday practice, what forces are pushing them to change and how they should adapt to those changes they wish to adopt.

The changes in Table 6.1 are slowly happening. Consultation time has lengthened (six and a half minutes to 10), surgeries have subsequently lengthened (one and a half hours to three hours), home visits have decreased in number, special clinics have multiplied (no longer just antenatal but diabetic, asthma and others), patients move about more and so on. All these factors impinge on communication and consultations, some in more subtle ways than others. (On a personal note, the main change in my way of working is that as I grow older I see patients more as partners than as passive recipients of health care.)

Consultation length

How did general practitioners manage to be patient centred in five minutes? Of course, doctors didn't unless the first five minutes was added to the next five-minute consultation and so on, so that at the end of the year a particular patient may have had 25 minutes or more of consultation time.

There are many reasons to increase consultation length. Research has shown that doctors with longer consultation times prescribe fewer drugs and offer more health promotion advice.[2] They are also more likely to explore psychosocial problems.[3] A group of eminent general practitioners, including a past president of the Royal College of General Practitioners, has identified five important influences on the content and thus the potential length of a consultation (Box 6.1).[4]

> **Box 6.1 ○ Influences on the content and length of consultations**
>
> ○ **Participatory consultation style** • patient-centred approach; exploring the patient's agenda; shared understanding; shared decision making.
>
> ○ **Extended professional agenda** • dealing with ongoing problems as well as presenting problems; health promotion; education.
>
> ○ **Access problems** • appointment systems; rising demand; availability of appointments.
>
> ○ **Loss of interpersonal continuity** • knowing or not knowing the doctor/patient well.
>
> ○ **Health Service reforms** • primary-care led NHS; primary care dealing with patients with more serious problems.

One size or length does not fit all. Not every illness and care-seeking behaviour can fit into a standard 10-minute box. Surgery times still overrun, due to patients' complex problems, but also due to interruptions, technical difficulties (computer malfunction) and difficulties focusing on priorities. While DNA (did not attend, i.e. missed their appointment) patients are annoying to staff, they do give the doctor a chance to catch up, or maybe even a break for a cup of coffee. There will probably never be an optimum consultation time. We can only hope for the best fit for the majority of patients.

In Australia many doctors offer routine 15-minute appointments. It certainly takes the pressure off to know that there is time for adequate discussion and explanation. The healthcare system is different though in that GPs may charge patients for consultations. The doctors who fund their practices solely through the state health insurance scheme, Medicare, often run five-minute appointments as standard. Patients reserve paying for the doctor's time when they feel they have a more complicated problem, rather than just wanting a prescription for antibiotics. For these complicated issues they will return to see the doctor they are more likely to consider their *own* doctor, which has implications for continuity of care.

Continuity of care

Older general practitioners speak longingly of the days when they knew all their patients and their patients knew them. It was a time when many GPs practised single-handedly and drugs were prescribed as the 'The Tablets. Take one four times a day.' Nowadays we speak of continuity of care and wonder about its passing. Doctors and patients move practices more freely, and there are walk-in clinics and more part-time GPs. What effect if any will this have on consultations and communication skills?

○ **Continuity of care** *care from one doctor, usually spanning an extended time and more than one episode of illness.*[5]

The above definition reflects that personal care of the GP for their personal list of patients. It assumes 24-hour care, seven days a week. This cosy picture of general practice would no longer be recognised by the younger generation of general practitioners, whose working day is much shorter, and who consider themselves as members of a primary care team. Today's continuity is more likely to be served by that team than by one individual.

Whether patients are best managed by one individual is a question that perhaps we should not seek to answer given that the 21st-century GP is no longer able or willing to follow the work patterns of their predecessors. From personal experience it is obviously quicker and more satisfying to consult with a patient over many years. Rather than think of single consultations of seven or 10 minutes, GPs considered the many interactions with that patient. Our experience was that consultations did not begin with a blank sheet (or empty computer screen) but rather a wealth of knowledge on both sides of the relationship built up painstakingly, including meetings at night and in the home, with the family and with the pets (crawling into the doctor's bag).

George Freeman, Professor of General Practice at the University of London, draws a distinction between longitudinal continuity of care and personal care (Box 6.2). He suggests that current evidence does not support the idea that it is better for patients to see only the same doctor for each consultation. However, he does feel that patients should be able to see the doctor of their choice as far as is practicable.[6] The distinction between the two types of continuity is subtle. Longitudinal care is only measured by time (quantity) rather than quality. A patient may be registered with the same doctor for many years but not feel completely happy with that doctor's interpersonal skills. However, changing doctors in the past was a more difficult business than it is today. Personal continuity assumes that the doctor has empathy and personal responsibility towards the patient rather than just a relationship built on the passage of time and number of contacts alone. Personal care improves communication and trust.[7]

Patients will often wait for some time to be able to see 'their own' doctor, whereas for other patients the priority is to be seen as soon as possible. When patients are asked what they perceive as quality of care they feel that seeing the same GP a lot of the time is an indicator.[8] Patients value a personal doctor–patient relationship, in particular for what they consider are

---

Box 6.2 ○ Continuity of care

Longitudinal continuity (care over time):

○ care given by one doctor over a defined time

○ usually a single-handed GP

○ evidence of benefit mainly from secondary-care out-patient settings.

Personal continuity (care of an individual patient):

○ ongoing therapeutic relationship between patient and doctor

○ patient looks to this doctor as most valued source of care

○ nature and quality of contacts more important than number.

---

more serious conditions, including those with psychological and/or family factors.[9] They define personal care as including good communication skills, they appreciate empathy and they prefer whole-patient or holistic care.[10] For complex problems patients want a doctor who is familiar with their family background and concerns, and they are prepared to wait to get this level of personal care.[10]

○ **Holism** *the integration of physical, psychological and social components of health problems in making diagnoses and planning management.[11]*

Ensuring longitudinal and personal care by having patients only see one doctor cannot now be sustained. Many GPs work part time within practices either because of reduced working hours or because of other commitments to service delivery such as committee membership, clinical governance or education. Equity of workload is important and GPs are usually happy to see patients with new problems or to manage patients with chronic disease even if they have not consulted with this patient before. However, patients with complicated medical histories, psychosocial intricacies and multiple unexplained symptoms should be encouraged to see the same doctor as much as possible so that a planned and agreed management plan may be carried out. If this is not possible, the medical record is an important instrument in ensuring quality of care as patients transfer between doctors. Patients may become accustomed to developing a relationship with a group of doctors,[12] perhaps each individual doctor–patient relationship being subtly different to meet that patient's needs at various times.

Loss of personal continuity may have other consequences. Doctors are less likely to find out the consequences of their diagnosis and management, find out the outcomes of their 'wait and see' decisions and follow an illness episode from start to finish. This lack of feedback could reduce the educational potential of consultations unless GPs specifically look up the sequelae of patient encounters over weeks and months. This process is even more difficult for doctors who practise mainly as locums, moving from surgery to surgery and rarely building up any significant doctor–patient relationships. Their approach to consultations may vary significantly from GP principals who grow with and learn from their communities. Locum GPs themselves have cited lack of patient follow-up as one negative feature of their role.[13]

Most patients understand the concept of the medical team. They realise that medical records are shared and often expect a GP to know all about them, even if this is the first time they have consulted with this individual. Patients have learned to book in for consultations with practice nurses without getting the doctor's permission first.

These factors have led to the definition of three other types of continuity (Box 6.3).[14] The passing of information between health professionals should

---

Box 6.3 ○ Three more types of continuity of care

Informational continuity

The use of information on past events and personal circumstances to make current care appropriate for each individual.

Management continuity

A consistent and coherent approach to the management of a health condition that is responsive to a patient's changing needs.

Relational continuity

An ongoing therapeutic relationship between a patient and one or more providers.

---

encompass more than medical history and treatment. But how should we archive the patient-centred approach of the initial consultation and subsequent meetings? How may a complex story complete with health beliefs, concerns and expectations be translated onto the computer screen so that the next interaction does not need to start from a position of ignorance on either side? Perhaps the patient choosing to see a different GP for an acute problem does not want that GP to know all the complexities of the previous story. That story should be reserved, perhaps, for the personal doctor.

Certainly management needs to be discussed between members of the team so that a logical plan is followed. Shared protocols and patient-held records improve the likelihood of treatment continuity. However, if the shared decision-making process has resulted in the patient's ultimate decision to choose a course of action at odds with accepted medical wisdom, this may not be acceptable to other team members. Conflict may arise. It is important that the team meets regularly to discuss practice philosophy and those patients with complex problems who, either by choice or through necessity, consult with more than one team member.

Walk-in centres

Nurse-led walk-in centres were introduced in the NHS in 1999. Their effect on patient care and issues relating to communication and continuity of care are still being assessed. The international experience shows that such centres are used primarily when other healthcare services are closed. Patients predominantly have minor illnesses and injuries; their satisfaction is high because they like the convenience of the centres.[15] Early results from the UK show similar results, with patients often attending on the first day of their illness and being less likely to want a prescription. Such patients are not concerned about continuity of care, but about one-third of them intend to attend their own general practice for follow-up. This means that GPs need to enquire about other information and advice given to patients and their source.[16] Little is known as yet about the quality of care and communication at these centres, and the impact they will have on the more traditional GP–patient relationship.

Quality of care

○ **Quality** *degree or grade of excellence; having a high degree of excellence.*

Doctors are expected to provide quality of care to patients. This is part of the National Health Service agenda. The document *A First Class Service: Quality in the New NHS*, published in 1998, lists one element of quality that is of direct interest to the consultation: 'involving patients in their own treatment and care' (5.9).[17] The main issues are defining quality and then measuring it. Researchers from the National Primary Care Research and Development Centre (NPCRDC) in Manchester have defined its components as a combination of access (whether patients can obtain health care) and the effectiveness of clinical and interpersonal care (whether the care is any good once accessed).[18]

Measuring quality is difficult. The length of consultations is one measure that has been used but this is only a proxy because what is important is obviously what goes on in the consultation. The NPCRDC team has used four outcome measures for quality: chronic disease management; preventative care; access and interpersonal care; and team climate and effectiveness. Each of these measures is scored based on criteria devised by a team of GPs who combined evidence with expert opinion. Four variables stood out as predictors of quality. The largest effect was indeed consultation length. The other three were size of practice, deprivation and team climate.[19]

Quality chronic disease management involves collecting data about patients (smoking status, blood pressure, action taken with regards to abnormal blood results such as lipid levels). It must also involve a measure of what the patient understands and how the patient has been involved in decisions. These interpersonal/communication outcomes are more difficult to quantify. Often it has to be assumed that such outcomes as changes in smoking status and increased uptake of lifestyle advice are related to good communication between doctor and patient.

Professor and GP John Howie and his team from Edinburgh have developed a 'consultation quality index' (CQI), which they believe reflects the core values of general practice. They use as proxies for these core values consultation length, how well the patients know the doctor and patient enablement.[20] The latter is discussed in Chapter 8. The UK GP contract introduced in 2004 has a Quality and Outcomes Framework (QoF) through which GPs may earn extra funding by improving the quality of care within their practices. The quality indicators for this financial reward are: the care of patients with specific illnesses; patient record management; communication with patients; and staff training. The recurring themes for quality are thus consultation length, continuity of care and interpersonal skills.

Cultural competency within the consultation

We live and work in a multicultural society. This is self-evident. While urban practices are likely to have a richer mix of patients with varying cultural backgrounds, no practice within the UK is likely to consist solely of patients whose first language is English. A simple change is that a receptionist should no longer ask for a patient's Christian name. This is not an appropriate question for many people, and the appropriateness cannot be gauged only by assumptions from the surname as to religion and background.

When considering communication the issues are not just about 'mother tongue' but also more subtle differences in social support, health beliefs, reli-

gious ideology and healthcare expectations. Historically doctors, who practised for many years in the same area even though they originally came from
a different region, would begin to understand their patients' health beliefs
as they worked and socialised within that area. However, the increasing
mobility of the population means that doctors are often ignorant of their
patients' backgrounds and beliefs. Exploring patients' ideas and concerns
is challenging if we assume that these will be similar to what we have met
before. In these circumstances empathy may be difficult. When communication is difficult because of a language barrier as well, how are we to help
these patients? Consultations become frustrating for both doctor and patient.
Such interactions have been labelled 'veterinary medicine' by some. This
disparaging way of thinking about GPs' work holds some truth, but we have
to overcome the barriers so that communication is possible on some level.

Cultural competency is an agreed core value for clinicians that is taught at
medical school and on postgraduate courses. The terms cultural awareness,
cultural sensitivity and multiculturalism are also used. Culture is used in a
broad sense to include diversity in cultural identity, race, ethnicity, religious
belief and sexual identity. We could also add social class or at least socio-economic standing, and physical or intellectual ability.

○ **Culture** *the totality of socially transmitted behaviour patterns, arts,*
beliefs, institutions and all other products of human work and thought; those
patterns, traits and products considered as the expression of a particular
period, class, community or population; those patterns, traits and products
considered with respect to a particular category, such as a field, subject
or mode of expression; the predominating attitudes and behaviour that
characterise the functioning of a group or organisation and the intellectual
and artistic activity and the works produced by it etc.

A reductionist view of cultural competency is to list the three domains of
learning (knowledge, skills and attitudes) and to evaluate performance in
each one. A doctor should know, for example, what contraception practices
are acceptable to practising Catholics or the arrangements after a Jewish
patient has died. Skills might include communicating with an Aboriginal
patient and accepting the lack of eye contact as a cultural norm. Attitudes
might be my insistence that I am not racist and that I treat all patients the
same regardless of colour or background. These are of course simplistic outcomes and such education usually assumes that the learner comes from
what is the norm: white, Western, First World, orthodox medical background. I can show I am culturally aware by using all my consultation skills
and patient-centred approach to interact with a traumatised refugee from

Afghanistan with a sore throat. But can I measure the best outcome of this consultation as a shared decision not to prescribe antibiotics? What is the best outcome for doctor and patient in this scenario, and how do we know?

Modern educational theory has moved on from looking at 'knowledge, skills and attitudes' to concepts of roles or competences; for successful completion of a specified task or role different aspects of medical competence need to be brought together. In this framework competence is defined as the ability to assume a combination of well-defined roles.[21] One such role is as provider of direct patient care including to people from different cultural backgrounds, i.e. cultural competency.

Cultural competency has been criticised as an attempt to inculcate into medical students and doctors the characteristics of each diverse group of patients, so that they can provide better health care because they will no longer hold ignorant or biased views about their patients.[22] However, the cookbook approach may reduce diversity to a simplistic level, presenting cultures as static rather than dynamic. It is easy to stereotype, to attribute to one person the characteristics of a whole group of people because of some similarities. However, within a culturally similar group there will be many differences. Two white male English-speaking 35-year-old patients living in the same street cannot be expected to have the same ideas, concerns and expectations. Neither can two Asian 35-year-old patients who may have very different backgrounds. A study of British Bangladeshi patients with diabetes found that their attitudes towards the condition were influenced not only by their cultural inheritance but also by their social circumstances and level of deprivation, attributes they shared with their non-Bangladeshi neighbours. Thus with regards to health beliefs in the two groups, the similarities were as striking as the differences.[23]

An unemployed Asian living in a tower block may have more in common with an unemployed white Londoner living in slum conditions than with an affluent Asian businessman. However, assumptions should never be made. Describing someone as 'white' is almost meaningless; the description is too broad. The doctor needs to go back to first principles and listen to the patient's story.

Doctors must learn to discover patients' identities that are not limited by a definition of their race, ethnicity or culture. In the postmodernist world of the early 21st century GPs need to acknowledge that these identities change over time. They are slippery due to the impact of new social movements, globalisation and racism.[24]

In the nursing field Leininger, the founder of the transcultural nursing movement in the USA, has described three possible modes of healthcare intervention.[25] Care oriented towards cultural preservation involves acknowledging a patient's cultural health beliefs and working with them in a complementary way with our own 'orthodox' views. Cultural negotiation means that both parties aim to understand the other's viewpoint and compromise where necessary to ensure the best outcome for the patient. Cultural repatterning is more difficult as it involves the health professional challenging a patient's way of life because it is unacceptable in the society in which we are living and practising. Examples of this would be British doctors refusing to perform female circumcision, which is now illegal, or attempting to intervene in some arranged marriages that are proving detrimental to the mental health of adolescent girls.

Macpherson (author of the Macpherson report into the murder of teenager Stephen Lawrence) has defined institutional racism as

> the collective failure of an organisation to provide an appropriate and professional service to people because of their colour, culture or ethnic origin. It can be seen or detected in processes, attitudes and behaviour which amount to discrimination through unwitting prejudice, ignorance, thoughtlessness and racist stereotyping which disadvantages minority ethnic people.[26]

Racism in society 'acts as a major hurdle to health and wealth'.[27] To avoid racism in the health service patients should be involved in service development. However, it is important to remember that discrimination may occur against doctors. Patients may make racist remarks against health service staff. A practice should have a policy that deals with such incidents.

Prejudice derives from many different sources. *The Integrated Threat Theory of Prejudice*, developed by US psychologists, suggests that prejudice arises from four interlinked conditions.[27] These have relevance to the consultation as shown on Table 6.2. However, one study from an educational setting showed that the strongest unique predictor of a person's attitude to people from different cultural or 'foreign' backgrounds is whether there is difficulty in communication. This difficulty could arise from accented speech, inability to speak each other's language or differences in non-verbal communication. Lack of communication then causes discomfort, impatience and frustration, leading to prejudice.[28]

Working with interpreters and patient advocates

Working in a multicultural health service means that GPs will often be conducting consultations with patients whose first language is not English. Doctor and patient need to consider whether such a consultation is feasible,

Table 6.2 ○ **Sources of prejudice**

Condition/source	Effect in a consultation
Negative stereotypes (cognitive beliefs)	Thinking of patients from different cultural backgrounds as lazy, arrogant, prone to psychosomatic complaints
Intergroup anxiety	Suspicious and hostile to outsiders; anxious and frustrated by an inability to understand each other and therefore help as a doctor
Realistic threats (economic and physical)	Believing that certain patients overuse NHS resources to which they have not contributed; a burden on the NHS
Symbolic/cultural threats	Patients undermine one's own culture and beliefs

SOURCE: Stephan W G and Stephan C W. Predicting prejudice. *International Journal of Intercultural Relations* 1996; **20**: 409–26.

depending on the extent of any language barrier. This may be difficult to assess, given that a patient may appear fairly fluent in English but may lack understanding of colloquialisms and technical terms, or jargon that the doctor uses. Checking understanding is therefore important.

Intercultural communication problems may lead to both high and low consultation rates within different groups of patients. Patients' lack of understanding may put them off seeing the same doctor again, or they may reattend frequently in search of meaning. To reduce communication difficulties patients prefer to register with a GP from their own ethnic group when possible.[29]

In certain circumstances doctor and patient may decide that an interpreter is needed. Interpreters should work in such a way that both effect and meaning of words and phrases are conveyed, and ideally should have relevant cultural knowledge and appropriate professional background.[30] Thus employing a family member as an interpreter is not recommended, though often this is an expedient solution to the problem of finding suitable interpreters. Even if a suitable interpreter is available there may be communication problems. Interpreters may subtly alter meaning, particularly when a patient's ideas and concerns, or less concrete concepts, are being discussed.

A patient-centred approach and shared decision making are difficult in such circumstances, and, with time constraints to be taken into account, it is understandable that a GP may revert to a more paternalistic style in such consultations. However, for all the reasons discussed in this book, this it not an ideal situation.

Patient advocates are becoming more common in health care. An advocate works on behalf of a patient to ensure that care is optimal and that there is good communication and shared understanding between the patient and health professionals. An advocate should not make decisions for a patient or express views as to which treatment option is best. An advocate should not have access to a patient's medical records and must be aware of their obligation to respect patient confidentiality. Sometimes advocates may work as interpreters as well but they should be trained to undertake this role. Health advocacy, as opposed to straightforward interpretation, may provide a useful way of bridging gaps in cultural understanding.

Issues relating to patients who are refugees and migrants

Voluntary migrants are people who have chosen to leave their own country and settle in a new place. Refugees, as defined by the United Nations, have left their home country due to a well-founded fear of persecution for reasons of race, religion, nationality, membership of a particular social group or political opinion. They are unable or unwilling to return home for fear of persecution. Refugees living in the UK while waiting for permission to stay in the country are called asylum seekers. As well as cultural concerns new arrivals to the UK or other host country may have anxieties relating to their immigration status and family separation, as well as marginalisation and discrimination. Key areas to be considered in consultations with these patients are shown in Box 6.4. As many refugees have stories of torture the doctor also needs to be aware of the effect of such consultations on himself or herself. The number of asylum seekers in the UK has dropped from about 20,000 per quarter year in 2002 to about 8000 per quarter in 2004, with the highest numbers being from Iran, China and Somalia.[31]

Social justice

Some of the problems that patients present with and that health professionals struggle to help them with have their roots in social deprivation and the inequality of modern society. With good communication skills health professionals elicit their stories of poor housing, lack of education, selfish neighbours and financial difficulties. Doctors' coping mechanisms may involve the diagnosis of depression and the prescribing of antidepressants even though they know that social factors are the main precipitants of the physical and psychological distress. Many GPs feel powerless in the face

> **Box 6.4** ○ **Consultations with refugees**
>
> ○ Ascertain their country of origin and reason for the move including immigration status.
>
> ○ Find out and be familiar with the context from which the patient has fled.
>
> ○ Is an interpreter needed?
>
> ○ What is the family situation? Do other members of the family need medical care?
>
> ○ Explore the patient's background and health beliefs in an open, non-discriminatory way.
>
> ○ Enquire about previous medical care including indigenous/non-Western approaches.
>
> ○ Explore stresses relating to the move and possible physical/mental abuse.
>
> ○ Is a patient advocate needed and available?
>
> ○ What social support is there?
>
> ○ Consider other needs besides medical ones. What help is available in these areas?

of social and health inequalities, and feel that they can only intervene on a personal, doctor–patient level.

Waitzkin writes:

> When a professional encourages mechanisms of coping and adjustment, this communication conveys a subtle political content. By seeking limited modifications, which preserve a particular institution's overall stability, the practitioner exerts a conservative political impact. Despite the best conscious intents the practitioner thus helps reproduce the same institutional structures that form the roots of personal anguish.[32]

Is it a GP's role to try to change society? What has this to do with consultation skills? We need to think about these issues as improvement in eliciting the patient's story and the realisation that the problem is not solely medical means that the shared management plan may involve 'treatment' other than medical or pharmacological. A criticism of enhanced communication skills and the recommendation to discover a patient's ideas and concerns is that health professionals will uncover problems that they cannot deal with. We all become uncomfortable with our powerlessness in the face of human misery. This is not a reason to go back to a purely medical history-taking framework. Professional duty also encompasses serving the greater society, and perhaps trying to deal with social injustice at some level.

Educational role of the GP: medical students and pre-registration house officers (PRHOs)

GPs are being asked to take an increasing role in the community-based education of undergraduate medical students. Medical students have a greater impact on a practice than a GP registrar, as they need observation and often sit in on consultations. This is bound to affect the dynamics of the doctor–patient interaction within the consultation. A questionnaire study from the Newcastle Medical School found that patients report learning more from consultations in which a student is present and they also feel they have more time to talk. However, 10 per cent stated they had left the consultation without saying what they wanted to say and about a third found it more difficult to talk about personal matters.[33] Such figures have implications for GPs who become involved in undergraduate education and who need to consider the impact of students on the quality of their consultations. However, teaching clinical skills has been shown to have a positive effect on the morale of GPs and to improve their own skills.[34]

Since 1999 in the UK, a small number of PRHOs (or interns) has been attached to general practices, on four-month rotation. In 2005 the structure of the first two years after qualification changed. The PRHO year is known as Foundation Year 1. The second year, or Foundation Year 2, includes a general practice attachment. PRHOs and Year 2 doctors have greater autonomy than medical students in that they are able to make management decisions and the GP tutor does not need to see every patient who consults with them. However, the GP tutor does need to be aware of the decisions and will need to sign any prescriptions, as PRHOs are not legally allowed to sign FP10s. Thus these consultations are likely to be seen as different by patients.

The impetus for the change towards more community- and primary care-based education of medical students arose first in the developing world,[35] with Europe and the USA also adopting a move towards a higher proportion of such education.[36] The reasons for this are well documented and include: changing patterns of healthcare delivery with reduced numbers of hospital in-patients;[37] recognition that patients in teaching hospitals are not representative of the general population;[38] and an emphasis on community management of chronic disease.[39]

In parallel with this more community-orientated approach to undergraduate education have been other developments in curriculum design. Since the acknowledgment of communication skills as a core competence for doctors,[40] medical students now spend more time learning and practising communication and consultation skills. Such skills are learnt well in primary care settings. GPs have a wealth of experience in learning and teaching consultation skills.[41] The move towards shared decision making also helps medical students understand the importance of this concept and is in line with the General Medical Council's (GMC) recommendations for undergraduate training. The GMC emphasises that doctors should be able to give information to patients in a way they can understand and fully involve patients in decisions about their care.[42] Hospital doctors are also undertaking communication skills training in greater numbers and communication is becoming an assessed competence for postgraduate qualifications such as those examined by the British royal colleges.

The changing nature of general practice ○ *reflections*

Like many GPs who have been in practice for 20 or more years I have experienced profound changes in the way my partners and I work. In my first practice after qualifying I was expected to consult at seven-minute intervals. Much later the 10-minute consultation became standard in the large group practice where I was a GP trainer. Now I enjoy the luxury of 15 minutes in Australia. I was able to see patients that quickly when I started work. I didn't like to keep them waiting and the stresses of getting behind, particularly on an on-call day, did not improve my health or my communication. I have now expanded to fill the allotted time. How can one share information and decisions in fewer than 15 minutes? Especially as now many doctors do not know their patients, have not built up a relationship over years. People move; doctors are less static. More of us are working part time in clinical work. Continuity is wonderful but difficult a lot of the time. Patients with diabetes attend special clinics and the doctor is not their 'regular'. Care is fragmented, but hopefully the diabetes is better controlled. I know the home conditions of very few patients. Our relationship is clinic bound. I moaned about home visits of course but I can certainly see their value.

We know about different countries and cultures from the television, the internet and our own travels. But this is on such a superficial level compared with that of communication about biopsychosocial problems. If we speak the same language we are lucky. Frustrations are felt on both sides. It once again comes down to time. I don't have the time to learn about all these patients. It is hard enough keeping up-to-date with medical advances without having to try to express myself in a different language or understand another health belief system. If our traditional role is changing, what will it be like in 10 years time? Will we be ready? Will we be satisfied?

○ Summary

- Patients value a personal doctor–patient relationship for what they consider are more serious conditions, including those with psychological and/or family factors.

- Consultation length is an important predictor of quality of care.

- Culture is used in a broad sense to include diversity in cultural identity, class, race, ethnicity, religious belief and sexual identity.

- Doctors must learn to discover patients' identities that are not limited by a definition of their race, class, ethnicity or culture.

- Interpreters should work in such a way that both effect and meaning of words and phrases are conveyed, and ideally should have relevant cultural knowledge and appropriate professional background.

REFERENCES

1 Willis J. *The Paradox of Progress*. Oxford: Radcliffe Medical Press, 1995, p. 107.

2 Deveugele M and Derese A. Longer consultations may be associated with improved outcomes in primary care. *Evidence-Based Healthcare* 2003; **7**: 75–6.

3 Howie J G R, Porter A M D, Heaney D J and Hopton J L. Long to short consultation ratio: a proxy measure of care for general practice. *BJGP* 1991; **41**: 48–54.

4 Freeman G K, Horder J P, Howie J G R, *et al*. Evolving general practice consultation in Britain: issues of length and content. *BMJ* 2002; **324**: 880–2.

5 Freeman G. Priority given by doctors to continuity of care. *Journal of the Royal College of General Practitioners* 1985; **5**: 423–6.

6 Freeman G and Hjortdahl P. What future for continuity of care in general practice? *BMJ* 1997; **314**: 1870.

7 McWhinney IR. Continuity of care in family practice. Part 2: Implications of continuity. *Journal of Family Practice* 1975; **2**: 373–4.

8 Bower P, Roland M, Campbell J and Mead N. Setting standards based on patients' views on access and continuity: secondary analysis of data from the general practice assessment survey. *BMJ* 2003; **326**: 258.

9 Kearley K E, Freeman G K and Heath A. An exploration of the value of the personal doctor–patient relationship in general practice. *BJGP* 2001; **51**: 712–18.

10 Tarrant C, Windridge K, Boulton M, Baker R and Freeman G. 'He treats you as a person not just a number.' How important is personal care in general practice? *BMJ* 2003; **326**: 1310–12.

11 Greenhalgh T and Eversley J. *Quality in General Practice: Towards a Holistic Approach.* London: King's Fund, 1999.

12 Davies P. The non-principal phenomenon: a threat to continuity of care and patient enablement. *BJGP* 2004; **54**: 731–2.

13 McKevitt C, Morgan M and Hudson M. Locum doctors in general practice: motivation and experiences. *BJGP* 1999; **49**: 519–21.

14 Haggerty J L, Reid R J, Freeman G K, Starfield B H, Adair C E and McKendry R. Continuity of care: a multidisciplinary review. *BMJ* 2003; **327**: 1219–21.

15 Salisbury C and Munro J. Walk-in centres in primary care: a review of the international literature. *BJGP* 2003; **53**: 53–9.

16 Salisbury C, Manku-Scott T, Moore L, Chalder M and Sharp D. Questionnaire survey of users of NHS walk-in centres: observational study. *BJGP* 2002; **52**: 554–60.

17 Department of Health. *A First Class Service: Quality in the New NHS.* London: Stationery Office, 1998.

18 Campbell S M, Roland M O and Buetow S. Defining quality of care. *Social Science and Medicine* 2000; **51**: 1611–25.

19 Campbell S M, Hann M, Hacker J, *et al.* Identifying predictors of high quality care in English general practice: observational study. *BMJ* 2001; **323**: 784–7.

20 Howie J G R, Heaney D J, Maxwell M, Walker J R and Freeman GK. Developing a 'consultation quality index' (CQI) for use in general practice. *Family Practice* 2000; **17**: 455–61.

21 Schuwirth L W T and van der Vleuten C P M. Changing education, changing assessment, changing research. *Medical Education* 2004; **38**: 805–12.

22 Wear D. Insurgent multiculturalism: rethinking how and why we teach culture in medical education. *Academic Medicine* 2003; **78**: 549–54.

23 Greenhalgh T, Helman C and Chowdhury M. Health beliefs and folk models of diabetes in British Bangladeshis: a qualitative study. *BMJ* 1998; **316**: 978–83.

24 Pfeffer N. Theories of race, ethnicity and culture. *BMJ* 1998; **317**: 1381–4.

25 Leininger M M. Cultural care diversity and universality. *Nursing Science Quarterly* 1988; **1**: 152–60.

26 Macpherson W. *The Stephen Lawrence Inquiry Report.* London: The Stationery Office, 1999.

27 Stephan W G and Stephan C W. Predicting prejudice. *International Journal of Intercultural Relations* 1996; **20**: 409–26.

28 Spencer-Rodgers J and McGovern T. Attitudes toward the culturally different: the role of intercultural communication barriers, affective responses, consensual stereotypes and perceived threat. *International Journal of Intercultural Relations* 2002; **26**: 609–31.

29 Arora S, Coker N and Gillam S. Racial discrimination in health services. In: Coker N (ed.) *Racism in Medicine*. London: King's Fund, 2001, pp. 141–67.

30 Robinson L. Intercultural communication in a therapeutic setting. In: Coker N (ed.) *Racism in Medicine*. London: King's Fund, 2001, pp. 191–210.

31 www.homeoffice.gov.uk/rds/pdfs04/asylumq204.pdf [accessed August 2006].

32 Waitzkin H. *The Politics of Medical Encounters*. New Haven: Yale University Press, 1991.

33 O'Flynn N, Spencer J and Jones R. Does teaching during a general practice consultation affect patient care? *BJGP* 1999; **49**: 7–9.

34 Hartley S, Macfarlane F, Gantley M and Murray E. Influence on general practitioners of teaching undergraduates: qualitative study of London general practitioner teachers. *BMJ* 1999; **319**: 1168–71.

35 World Federation for Medical Education. The Edinburgh Declaration. *Medical Education* 1988; **22**: 481–2.

36 Boaden N and Bligh J. *Community-Based Medical Education*. London: Arnold, 1999, pp. 29–41.

37 Institute for the Future. *Health and Health Care, 2010, the Forecast, the Future, the Challenge*. San Francisco: Jossey-Bass, 2000, pp. 6–8.

38 Green L A, Fryer G R Jr, Yawn BP, Lanier D and Dovey S. The ecology of medical care revisited. *New England Journal of Medicine* 2001; **344**: 2012–25.

39 Secretaries of State for Health, Wales, Northern Ireland, and Scotland. *Working for Patients*. London: HMSO, 1989.

40 World Health Organization. *Doctor–Patient Interactions and Communication*. Geneva: WHO, 1993.

41 Whitehouse C R. The teaching of communication skills in UK medical schools. *Medical Education* 1991; **25**: 311–18.

42 General Medical Council. *Duties of a Doctor*. London: GMC, 1995.

Preparing for patients in the 21st century

Learning to listen and to engage

This chapter explores:

- how changing realities of the professional patient/relationship affect developing ethical and effective communication • the evolution of consultation skills learning • valuing the patient perspective
- listening and responding to learners • learning to listen and to engage – examples and methods • principles of learning how to consult effectively • reflective practice and helping people make changes • helping learners in difficulty • the learning environment and resources.

'Where Osler could treat patients as passive consumers of care which doctors devised and nurses implemented, but patients unquestioningly endured, we must accept patients as colleagues in a jointly designed and performed production, in which they will nearly always have to do most of the work.'

JULIAN TUTOR HART, 1988
a retired GP who previously practised in South Wales; this influential writer and GP researcher coined the phrase 'the inverse care law' [1]

'Do not confine children to your own learning for they were born in another time.'

HEBREW PROVERB

How can professionals learn to be in partnership with patients for the 21st century? We do not (cannot) know all 'the answers', as they will be developed afresh during every encounter with patients and learners, but we offer some evidence and insights from experience and research. This chapter returns to some of the themes of earlier chapters in more detail. It provides histories and examples of doctors learning to talk, and work, with patients.

Changing realities and perceptions

The boundaries of the roles and relationship of doctor and patient are shifting constantly. Health economic policies mean that professionals' roles are being redefined, often in order to contain costs. Recruitment and retention of doctors is also a concern in a world where many want more variability in their working lives and flexibility to lead a broader life with space for family and personal interests. In the UK there are radical changes in the deployment of GPs, with more becoming freelance or salaried doctors employed by GP partnerships and healthcare trusts. Aspects of the doctor's role in primary care are being devolved to other professions, while some specialist medical tasks are now being undertaken by GPs.

We have already mentioned some of the changes in consultation practice resulting from the move from long-term GP relationships with patients to more short-term encounters that often involve other health professionals, as well as aspects of the targets of the present GP contract that appear to hinder communication.

Patients', health professionals' and policy makers' views of the relationship between doctors and patients have also evolved as health care has changed. The growth of patient and voluntary groups in health, the diverse information available about healthy living, sickness and cures, the greater questioning of authority figures and the growth of consumerism, mean that many patients now think and behave differently, and have varying expectations of professionals. The General Medical Council (GMC) and the royal colleges in the UK have responded to public anxieties about the misuse of doctors' power and have opened up to accountability. *The Patient's Charter* of 1991 defined the rights of patients and the standards of service they should expect within the NHS.[2] The Conservatives' white paper of 1989, *Working for Patients*, ensured that medical audit was introduced.[3] The Labour government has advocated increased patient choice within the health service.[4] NHS policy also now calls for active involvement of patients and communities as another route to reducing demand on services while improving public health.[5] Such a community development approach with its emphasis on shared responsibility has been promoted across continents with European, American and Australasian health communities learning from the wider world.[6]

We can only guess at the new social order for later 21st-century primary care professionals. Preparing GP registrars and others successfully for interacting with patients will have to involve the development of their capacities to deal with change and difference, and their ability to collaborate.[7]

This 'radical change in professional and public roles'[8] has profound consequences for the balance of power in meetings between patients and professionals. We have discussed the move from notions of paternalism to partnership in the consultation; other ways of conceiving of an equal 'meeting between experts'[9] for the 21st century include GP Julian Tudor Hart's description of patients and GPs making decisions together about their health service in the context of available resources.[1] Muir Gray (Director of the NHS National Electronic Library for Health and Public Health) has described the resourceful patient as someone who is supported to command inner personal and external resources for their healing, including internet access to information before, during and after consultations with professionals.[10] Angela Coulter (Chief Executive of the Picker Institute, which promotes patient-centred care) talks of the autonomous patient who is in ultimate charge of their healing process and decisions.[11] John Launer's (GP, based at the Tavistock Clinic, London) narrative approach 'places practitioners and patients on a more level footing, in a way that is more consistent with a contemporary understanding of patients' rights and professionals' duties'.[12]

As patients are now encouraged to tell us, their illness journey involves encounters with many kinds of people, only some of whom are professionals. The DIPEx (database of patient experiences of health and illness) website, for example, contains patients' personal experiences of health and illness, which they wish to share with others so that patients and health professionals may learn from these.[13] Doctors are only one kind of professional involved with patients, albeit at times the most powerful. Learning to link their medical contribution to a patient's healing with the personal work of patients, their families, friends and communities, and the professional work of nurses, therapists and other colleagues, is at the core of the GP's personal, professional task. It can be said to be about helping patients do their own healing work.[12, 14] For example, a practice in London's East End has the ethos of being a healthy learning community, working in partnership with local people, communities and primary healthcare teams to support the development and growth of individuals and leaders.[15]

As anyone who works with first-year medical students knows, the long-standing image of the doctor as powerful healer and society leader can sit uneasily with these notions of partnership with patients, and the importance and/or prospect of working in a team. Medical students tend to be very anxious about the huge responsibilities they feel will soon be theirs, and are often confused about the limits of these responsibilities and of their authority.[16] Some students in their early years overestimate both what is required of them and their own capacities to meet such demands, behaving with an arrogance that belies their underlying lack of confidence. Other students find the recent media attention to doctors' deficits demoralising, and sometimes react defensively. Even experienced GPs can feel that recognising the patient's contribution will mean that their own hard-earned skills and expertise are disparaged.[17] Yet we need our doctors to be healers, not mere medical mechanics in the team, and we need them to realise the power they have for this. Despite the growing evidence that listening to patients and enabling them to be fully engaged with solving problems actually promotes healing,[18] doctors often still find it hard to do.

Like others,[19] we have found that from early on in their working lives doctors learn to stop listening as a defence against the perceived burden of patients' pain.[20,21] We know that many newly qualified GPs in the UK cannot demonstrate listening to patients and working with their ideas,[22] despite having received consultation skills teaching about patient-centred medicine in their vocational training. Research suggests that UK patients are more likely than not to be treated in a paternalistic fashion in primary care with little shared decision making,[23] as we discuss more fully in Chapter 3. There are implications for policy makers about the external forces that shape practitioners' behaviour in consultations and for educationalists about interventions needed to support changes in their behaviour.

In the rest of this chapter we shall explore, through history, observations, stories and examples of learning and development, how communication and consultation skills learning has recently evolved: why there have been, and still are, difficulties with a partnership model; and what helps professionals learn to listen and work with patients.

Learning from the 20th century: the evolution of the learning and teaching of consultation skills

We have already outlined the development of the consultation from early times. The development of ways of learning how to consult has happened during our lifetimes. During the 20th century, partnerships between doctors and others from different traditions have looked to marry the art and science of healing in modern health care. Sociologists, psychologists, patients, patient advocates, carers, artists, educationalists, philosophers, other health professionals and, increasingly, policy and business analysts, have contributed to a wider understanding of the doctor–patient relationship. These different ways of seeing have resulted in debates about the purposes of communication in health care and how we should study, practise and teach it. Deeper approaches that develop understanding of the complexity of human relationships and healing have been contrasted to reductionist and surface approaches to performance in communication skills.[24] There have been calls to integrate communication and clinical skills teaching, rather than students learning these as separate entities (we describe the value of integrating these during assessment in Chapter 8).[25] In the following history and examples, we demonstrate and explore our growing understanding of the ways in which students, trainees, registrars and practitioners are best supported to help patients. Like others, we always say 'there is no one right way to communicate'. At the heart of the matter are questions of how we value others and think we can help them.

Valuing the patient perspective: developing a method

The largest group of active, non-medical contributors to current teaching about communication is simulated patients (SPs). Many people from local communities now work with medical and other health professional schools, and within postgraduate teaching and assessment centres in the UK, North America, Europe and Australasia.

A core site for the development of SPs in the UK in the late 1970s and early 1980s was the Department of General Practice at Manchester University. The study of British GP consultations by Byrne and Long (GP and professor, and sociologist respectively) had provided a basis for the first definitions of 'doctor-centred' and 'patient-centred' consultations.[26] Simply, in a minority of the consultations studied, patients had a voice; they literally had more of a say in the focus and content of the consultation.

The department served a deprived community. Early work by the general practitioner Bain, analysing his own consultations, had pointed to the greater lack of involvement in medical consultations of patients with lower socio-economic status.[27] This continues to be a source of inequity[28] and a major concern for developers of medical communication. When David Metcalfe followed Byrne as professor, he looked for ways to help medical students include the voice and wider world of patients during interviews. Metcalfe invited a local community theatre company 'North West Spanner' to work with him.[29]

The core values and research of the department encouraged a partnership approach to learning from others. The teaching benefited from the theatre company's understanding of communication and creative learning in groups in the local community. The company moved on from role-playing patients, as an audio-visual aid to doctors' ideas, to becoming teachers in their own right. The company accomplished this by helping to develop the roles and method of feedback, so that the scenarios were more authentic and were able to be sustained during feedback and when working through different approaches. They thus provided a lay patient voice in patient-centred, experiential learning for medical students.[30]

This method was later extended with David Pendleton, the psychologist, and his GP colleagues (authors of the seminal work *The Consultation: An Approach to Learning and Teaching*) to vocational training of general practitioners[31] and with nurses and GPs in professional development.[32,33,34] The method has since been developed in wider work with patients as teachers,[35] and with the professional development of midwives.[36] How an effective patient voice is developed in SP teaching and beyond is explored further in Chapter 9.

Listening and responding to learners: developing a method

North West Spanner (later known as Spanner Workshops) had begun its drama work in one of the poorest area of the UK, reminiscent of conditions described in the 19th century.[37] The ideas and practice of the young theatre company were influenced by living and working amongst the families who survived and flourished, often against many odds, in the transition from the debris of abandoned, terraced streets to high-rise developments.

Brazilian educator Paulo Freire (1921–97), who championed the oppressed, was one of the most influential thinkers about education in the 20th century.[38] His ideas help to explain the approach the group brought to changing communication in medicine. Freire described how poor peasants, urban dwellers and middle-class students in Brazil in the 1960s developed a 'problem-posing' form of learning to satisfy their need to make a difference to their world, as opposed to a 'banking' concept of education. In this model, people generated both questions and answers from their own, shared capabilities, rather than the traditional notion of learners as individual, empty vessels having expertise poured into them by their teachers. They broke out of a 'culture of silence' to talk together to deal critically with their reality.

Listening to learners and working from their needs – a learner-centred approach – are now established principles in medical education, particularly communication learning,[39] although adhering to these can be a struggle. The challenge for learners and teachers includes what Freire describes as the 'fear of freedom', or fear of the unknown.[38] Searching for the comfort and containment of certainty, students seek simple answers. Teachers, sometimes anxious to protect their status and usually anxious to do their job well, find it hard to trust that learners have the capacity to change, and, moreover, that they alone have that capacity, i.e. some of it is unknown to the teacher. Learners need to create their new ways of seeing the world in dialogue with each other. Most recently, this notion has been explored in writing about 'communities of practice'.[40]

○ **Postmodernism** *the rejection of universal stories and conventional philosophy, allowing different interpretation through individual perception; there is no one truth.*

Now postmodern notions of epistemology (the nature of knowledge) and understanding in medicine permeate education guidelines and curriculum design; medicine especially is not a set body of knowledge. Therefore students and their teachers have to learn how to keep learning.

The form of this early UK general practice teaching – well facilitated, small-group, reflective discussion of role plays with SPs, watched through a two-way screen – lent itself to creative learning. Like Freire, the members of Spanner brought to their educational work a conviction, supported by experience, that ordinary people as well as young students could choose their own way forward. So they respected the students' capacities to change. They role-played patients with the same respect and integrity, and, increasingly, were recruited from the local community. In reflective dialogue with a patient voice and their peers, students explored wider ways of understanding and behaving with patients.

This is far from a notion of standardising patients and ways to respond to them, of creating lists of defining behaviours, of attempting to capture a comfort zone of 'how to do it'. At the time, Manchester general practice could be said to exemplify a creative approach, open to patient and learner perspectives, while earlier communication skills courses involved teaching sets of skills to 'manage' patients. It was in general practice, with the work of David Tuckett *et al.*[9] (a team of sociologists based in Cambridge; see also Chapters 2 and 9) and David Pendleton *et al.*,[31] that the patient's ideas and concerns were made central.

There follow reports of experiments and examples of experiential and work-based learning of communication skills, to inform our model for preparing for patients in the 21st century.

Learning to listen and to engage

Example 1 – a controlled trial
In 1986 Penny Morris became the first full-time, designated teacher of communication in a British medical school, as a research/teaching fellow at Cambridge. This represented a major opportunity to develop and evaluate communication skills teaching across the clinical specialities, not only in general practice and psychiatry. Previous studies, mainly in North America, had shown that it was possible to improve medical students' abilities to com-

municate. In 1986, a British study was published which showed that training in collecting information from patients resulted in improvements that
persisted over time; however, both experimental and control groups performed badly at information giving, i.e. the 'second half' of the consultation,
referred to in Chapters 3 and 4.[41]

The particular impetus for the Cambridge post was the issuing of guidelines by the GMC.[42] For the first time, training in communication skills
throughout the undergraduate medical curriculum was recommended.
Richard Wakeford, in his survey of medical schools, had found that no medical school in the UK had more than minimal training in the collecting and
giving of information, and most schools offered nothing.[43] There was thus a
need for the assessment of the effect of a substantial attempt to teach these
skills.[44]

The model for this research was based on what had so far been understood
from the study of consultations in UK general practice and US general medicine: explanation must be clear, but responsive to what is on the patient's
mind. The tasks of negotiating based on shared understanding were emphasised, rather than a concentration on particular behaviours only, as had been
the case with most other rating approaches.[43] However, specific communication skills – particularly in structuring and listening – that had been shown
to facilitate patients expressing themselves[45] were also explored.

The rating scale (Oxbridge Rating Scale) used to evaluate the teaching
reflected this approach (Table 7.1), building on the work of Pendleton et
al.[31] This scale was developed with Theo Schofield and the other assessors
involved in the study, most of whom were examiners for the Royal College
of General Practitioners (RCGP). Previous evaluation methods had stressed
'eye contact' and 'expressions of empathy' at the expense of emphasising
that the task of the consultation was to share understanding, decisions and
care with the patient, and that various skills may be used to that end. This
method sought to redress the tendency for doctors to use communication
skills for manipulating a 'hidden agenda' from patients or for 'managing'
patients who may cause professionals difficulty, i.e. silencing them; rather,
the aim was to encourage a transparent structure, a shared agenda and an
activated patient.

Students at Cambridge work in small supervision groups during their
clinical years. The research/teaching fellow worked with half of the groups
and their clinical supervisors, providing, in particular, opportunities for
practice with simulated patients, trained by Spanner Workshops, who gave
individual feedback. Evaluation showed that these experimental students
performed all the above tasks better than the students in the control group,
who had received the standard clinical skills teaching only.

Table 7.1 ○ **Oxbridge Rating Scale of P Morris and T Schofield**[44]

	1	**2**	**3**	**4**	**5**
1 History: elicits the patient's history and symptoms, chronology and related factors sufficiently to establish the possible causes					
2 Question style: demonstrates the appropriate use of open, closed and reflective questions					
3 Structuring: conducts the consultation in a sequence logical to that particular patient's needs, and lets the patient know and follow the sequence, so that time is used effectively					
4 Listening: listens to the patient and responds to offers					
5 Patient's understanding and ideas: explores the patient's understanding and ideas about the nature and cause of the problems, and their management					
6 Patient's worries and concerns: explores and responds to the patient's worries and concerns about the problems, and their management					
7 Explaining: offers an appropriate explanation to the patient of the problems and their management that is related to the patient's own ideas					
8 Checking: checks that the patient understands any explanations and that concerns have been addressed					
9 Involving: takes opportunities to involve the patient in the decision making and their own management					
10 Relationship: establishes an effective relationship with the patient and demonstrates respect for the patient as a person					

RATED: 1 = unacceptable − 5 = very good.

This study developed and subsequently established effective and reliable methods for the teaching and evaluation of communication skills, particularly information-giving skills. Working with local clinicians helped develop awareness of the why and how of communication training, as did involving opinion leaders in developing the assessment instruments. The process of the research was thus used to help influence change, and the results contributed to movements to improve doctor–patient communication. Key principles learnt from this study related to teaching communication are shown in Box 7.1.

Further consultation research has supported the notion that what works best in improving health outcomes is the activation of patients.[46]

Box 7.1 ○ Principles of good communication skills teaching

① Teaching should occur alongside and with clinical teachers as far as possible, to help ensure that communicating well with patients is seen as an essential part of good medicine and not just an optional extra.

② Communication skills learning should be integrated with learning the tasks of the clinical consultation.

③ The timing of the teaching should reflect where learners are in their training.

④ Learners should be able to observe each other and reflect on their own practice of communicating with patients and, when working with SPs, the SPs should be similar to the patients they are seeing in their daily practice.

⑤ The method of practice and giving feedback should mirror the consulting style being taught, i.e. activating and involving. Learners are enabled to build on their strengths to learn specific approaches that suit them.

⑥ Learners should learn from a patient voice. This input is particularly valuable when learners have difficulties.

Gradually, the teaching of communication skills was becoming more prevalent in medical schools in the UK. GPs and others were starting to develop work with hospital clinical teachers so that history-taking teaching included communication skills. Meanwhile, further development work on overcoming barriers to listening to patients was needed.

Learning to listen and engage

Example 2 – Preparing for Patients

While watching working clinicians consult with patients, real and simulated, it became clearer that doctors often chose to ignore patients' cues, rather than that they had missed them. This seems to some of us in the communication skills field to be about how doctors deal with feelings. Unable to cope with their difficult feelings, doctors stop listening to patients, in part because they feel overwhelmed with responsibility. Balint groups, in which doctors reflect together on patients who trouble them and use the evidence of their own feelings to try to understand their patients better, flourished in the 1960s and 1970s, and have been revived in the last decade.[47] More behaviour-based approaches were later favoured, considered more likely to appeal to the hospital specialists whom communication skills advocates were trying to win over. An opportunity to explore how best to support doctors and students with difficult feelings arose when, as part of the next wave of pressure on medical schools to change their approach, resources were offered to innovate curriculum change. It was decided to develop a way for the medical science students at Cambridge to have some early personal and professional development as fledgling doctors who need to relate to patients.

A series of pilot courses were held, called 'Preparing for Patients'.[48] Collaborators included GPs experienced in the Balint tradition. These courses were evaluated and qualitative analysis carried out to examine what made them successful.[19]

The aim was to provide the core of a coherent learning structure to support medical students to cope with difficult feelings and thereby remain open to patients' concerns. The structure was based on the elements already described: a capacity-building model for doctor/patient and teacher/ student interactions. This included attention to safe groups for students to approach difficult situations, like their first interview with a patient. Students then moved on to more challenging tasks, always in a supportive environment. Active SPs were included and also patients as teachers, who could help reassure students that patients have the capacity to be involved in the discussion of care and share the burden. The local hospice provided opportunities for the students to experience confronting thoughts of pain, loss and death. Careful preparation for, and debriefing from, their experiences enabled structured reflection and built confidence. They could thus learn early on about the strengths of patients and relatives when in extremity, as well as develop understanding about how to help with their vulnerabilities. The idea was that students could develop a parallel understanding of patients' experience of illness and personal strategies for dealing with difficulties.

Personal and Professional Development (PPD) courses are now held in all UK medical schools, most of which provide more early contact with patients. There is variable emphasis on emotional support, depending on the teachers' conviction of its need and the availability of small-group work. Successful group work includes discussion of their current, important experiences, so that they can develop as learning groups where attitudes and values can be explored. Such groups continue in primary care, to support GPs throughout their working lives.[49]

These next case studies are about the learning experiences of practising GPs, who have given permission for their inclusion here.

Learning to listen and to engage

Example 3 – work-based learning using video

During this period, pressure on general practice had increased to the extent that retention to the profession became an issue.[50] Self-directed and practice-based learning groups were established to provide some sort of peer support. Groups of GPs reviewed their everyday work, often on video.[14] The following case study describes a piece of related work in London in 1998, building on the method that had been developed in Manchester and Cambridge.

Dr F started working as a GP in England in her early thirties. She had trained abroad and had worked as a hospital specialist. She underwent vocational training for general practice in England. She then practised in an inner-city partnership with a multi-ethnic population. She was interested in becoming more involved with education, like the partners in her practice.

She took the RCGP membership examination as part of her development as an educator, but failed the video assessment. The process of this assessment is rigorous and was rightly perceived as daunting since doctors must submit selected videos of their actual consultations with minute-by-minute self-analysis.

She reviewed her examination tape with an expert clinical assessor to ensure that she had not failed because of clinical error. I was asked to help her with her consultation skills, and funding for this work was obtained from the local health authority.

We reviewed videotapes of her consultations with patients. Failure to pass the consultation skill part of the membership video assessment usually meant that nothing was demonstrated in terms of involving patients in any way in problem setting and solving (personal communication, Peter Tate). Dr F agreed that her tapes contained no such evidence of patient involvement.

I encouraged her to identify her strengths, exploring with her the notion that to change she needed to build from what she could do well.

She managed a large range of complex patient cases, often with more than one person, while maintaining politeness, calm and attention. Many patients knew her and were relaxed with her. Some were quite new to the country, being refugees and often traumatised. She empathised with them as outsiders like herself. Many consultations required interpreters; there were a lot of patients waiting to be seen without appointments and the surgery was always packed, despite many doctors and consulting rooms, and long hours. (One of our sessions was held at her surgery premises so that I could witness her challenges.)

Dr F did ask questions about her patients' social situations. She construed this as being patient centred and assumed that both the assessors and I would want her to delve more deeply into patients' circumstances. Rather, she needed help to see the point of *eliciting patients' reflections about the problems they had brought to her.* It was a revelation to Dr F that involving patients entails enabling patients to do more of their own work in facing and solving problems. It does not mean going into personal matters as a diagnostician or problem solver, for which GPs are no more equipped than any other person (and arguably less so than a member of the patient's immediate community).

She was not alone in this misconstruing of her role. Many registrars and practising GPs demonstrate similar confusion during video review. In primary care, doctors are faced with patients in their wider social and psychological world. The disease-centred, doctor-led model of much hospital practice is unhelpful for grappling with much of this. Doctors can then struggle with a sense of the limits of their own authority in dealing with patients' problems in the patients' own contexts.

What Dr F had taken from her experience of GP vocational training was a feeling of an overwhelming burden of patients' psychosocial issues that she should investigate and take on. Given her workload, she had in some sense chosen not to engage with any part of the patient's perspective.

Dr F was not used to reflective learning that respected her experience and feelings. She wanted me simply to tell her what to do. This is a common feature of some doctors' learning, often stemming from their previous undergraduate learning experiences during which they were used to being 'spoon fed' knowledge. Trying to develop patient-centred behaviours whilst still in a doctor-directed and teacher-directed framework can be counter-productive. Helping doctors to do their own reflective work on practice offers a model of respecting and working with others' experiences.

The process of doctors learning to do their own work of building on strengths to face change can help them to do the same for their patients. Doctors' work with patients then becomes more about supporting patients' own efforts to deal with their thoughts and feelings about their situation, rather than thinking they need to solve patients' psychosocial issues. We have found that, without the experience of being supported to learn for themselves, doctors wanting to be told what to do usually feel that their patients will want the same.

As well as our one-to-one sessions, Dr F had the opportunity to be involved in group work in her locality where GPs helped each other to review their consultations, using this approach.[51] In this setting, she was able to learn from others' examples and by helping them in the group work. The group also acknowledged the stresses of her working situation (it included another GP from her practice) and recognised her developing skills.

She has become more confident in showing her own videos to groups and to model learning from this. She testifies to and demonstrates the change in her approach to working with patients. She passed her subsequent video assessment and is now an active member of her local educational network.

These last two examples of helping those facing difficulty, whether as beginning students or as experienced practitioners, provide further guidelines for good teaching (Box 7.2).

Box 7.2 ○ Helping learners in difficulty

① Acknowledge difficulties.

② Respect learners' experiences.

③ Help them recognise their strengths.

④ Provide a supportive structure where learners explore problems and move on.

⑤ Encourage joining supportive groups.

The principle of working from where learners are applies also to experiential learning with experienced practitioners. In the 1990s, others found this too.[51] The following example illustrates how simulated patients can contribute to such learning.

Learning to listen and to engage

Example 4 – experiential learning with simulated patients
This interaction and debrief took place during a workshop at Leeds Medical School. Senior doctors were invited to attend workshops on teaching communication and consultation skills. Initial workshops were kept to three hours to make it possible for busy doctors from a variety of specialities to join in. The aim is to develop a community of practice where personal and professional skills, attitudes and context can be reviewed frankly in a solid framework, informed by a patient voice. They used the Spanner method described earlier, based on doctors' everyday work experience. The SPs were members of local patient and carer groups, trained by Spanner Workshops.

First, we established participants' objectives for the session and a structure for debriefing and feedback. Then two participants worked with the group to practise and review a simulated consultation, created on the spot to fit their daily practice.

Dr D was a young GP who came to the group because she wanted to help students with their consultation skills in a more structured manner. With the group, she first observed an Accident and Emergency consultant interview a young woman who had taken a paracetamol overdose. The consultant had wanted help with preserving his humane approach while under great pressure. The consultant demonstrated considerable skill and flexibility to try new approaches, despite feelings of impatience with self-inflicted injury. For him, the issue was time: he felt the eight minutes he spent talking with this woman was time he could barely spare in real life, pressured by his other, more technical responsibilities. The feedback from the SP role-playing the young woman powerfully emphasised the value of his careful discussion with her, both emotionally and technically, as she felt able to follow his clinical recommendations. Dr D was able to contribute a comment from her experience from general practice of the judicious use of time spent on the patient's perspective and how it can yield much in a little while. In her context, too, technical responsibilities were growing with targets for health promotion needing to be met.

Dr D then chose to work on 'something not straightforward that will need me to pay attention and include the targets'. An SP teacher chose a role she had already played in similar sessions: a woman presenting with what she called premenstrual tension (PMT). It is important that the doctor can be herself in the role-play as far as possible. So that Dr D would not have to pretend to know the 'patient', the SP decided to role-play as a relatively new patient who had not met this doctor before.

Dr D demonstrated a very effective, time-efficient exploration of the problem and the patient's perceptions. With the help of the group and the SP, still in role as the patient, she identified the following strengths of her consultation: she gave space ('Tell me … mmm … mmm'); clarified ('Can we look at this in a bit more detail?'); responded to and widened the patient's focus on her family ('How are they … with this?'), and on the patient's own efforts to improve things ('You say … how about … what's stopping you?'); and affirmed her position with an empathic statement ('You're a busy lady with a lot on your plate'). She explored the patient's ideas and summarised possible causes and solutions, including taking a blood test to assess hormone levels, finding more time to relax, and taking extra vitamins and antidepressants. She mentioned her information sheet on PMT. She reminded the patient about her cervical smear. Patient and doctor decided together that the patient would have a blood test, try to keep up her efforts to deal with stress with exercise, record the ups and downs of her moods, and come back for her smear and blood test result. This all took place in 10 minutes.

Dr D then examined a particular aspect of the consultation. She was concerned with the patient's management: she thought that many patients presenting like this were depressed and may need antidepressants, which they resist. The SP indicated that taking antidepressants would suggest that she had a fault line where she could not cope. This was the point of change for Dr D. The facilitator and SP did not suggest what she should do and the group held back their ideas. She was encouraged to reflect critically on the situation and her difficulties with it. She reflected that she herself was reluctant to prescribe, particularly as GPs' over-prescribing of antidepressants had been recently strongly criticised. She also felt a lot of empathy with the load this patient carried – a job and children. She thought the patient needed ways to find more time for herself and to share her burden.

She then retried the last part of the consultation with the SP, sharing her ideas more explicitly. Dr D mentioned depression, and, hearing the patient's resistance to this possible diagnosis and antidepressant treatment, invited her to consider ways that she, the patient, could lessen the stresses upon her. The patient thought she would talk to her husband about the ideas that had come up and how he, or others, could help.

With feedback from the SP and others, Dr D was enabled to explore alternatives and realised that she did have more to offer than antidepressants. It was acceptable to be more personal with patients and to bring their shared life experience to bear as an alternative to medication while helping manage problems of everyday life. As the lead for mental health in her practice, she now had insight to offer the meeting she had called to discuss their antidepressant prescribing.

She was also more confident to teach. Her previous experience of working with an SP had been in an unsafe structure and she had been feeling unconfident.

Example 4 supports recent findings that clinicians need to find ways to talk differently with patients about sharing understanding and decisions about treatment. As Muir Gray points out, the future clinician could become a 'knowledge manager' who can:

1. ask the right question and find possible answers

2. help the patient interpret the knowledge he or she has been given or has found for herself or himself.[10]

Work-based learning with a patient perspective can help professionals develop new approaches in clinical encounters with patients. This example illustrates the importance of working with 'real' material drawn from participants' encounters with patients and of providing safe structures so that professionals can explore real feelings. It also shows the importance of working with SPs who are authentic, convincing and can provide a voice to patients who may be stereotyped by professional perceptions. They help doctors believe that a partnership approach can be fruitful. This is further explored in Chapter 9.

The learning environment

GPs in practice now contend with a sense of pressure to include other factors in the consultation, apart from what brought the patient to the doctor. Like medical students trying to remember questions to analyse symptoms, they have to hold a number of agendas in mind, while paying attention to the patient. GPs are learning to cope with record keeping on computers in the consulting room, just as students struggle with taking notes for records while interviewing patients.

Balancing clinical tasks while working with patients is more complex in modern general practice, where GPs and patients come from increasingly diverse backgrounds. Research by Val Wass (Professor of Community-Based Medical Education at the University of Manchester) and others into GP and medical student consultations[52] suggests that we need to think of fresh ways to learn for such diversity in practice, which is explored in Chapter 9. Developing the capacity for self-awareness is the key to understanding and working with others. We have described some ways to support learners to develop self-awareness but it is a relatively neglected area in medical education so far. A core curriculum for communication in medical education drawn up by a group of teachers in the UK now acknowledges the need for attention to 'self awareness and survival'.[53]

Individual, reflective practice can help practitioners at all stages of learning to develop self-awareness and survival skills. This can be done by simply logging questions/doubts/needs that arise day by day during consultations with patients, then looking for opportunities to address these, while reading, on the internet or in discussions with colleagues.

The examples above illustrate how practising GPs as well as those in education and training can develop their consultation skills with others, throughout their career. Further resources that learners we work with have found especially helpful are:

- *Work Based Learning in Primary Care* – a journal that encourages self-directed learning (www.radcliffe-oxford.com/journals)

- www.bmjlearning.com – with online learning exercises and record keeping

- www.besttreatments.co.uk – for your patients

- *The Doctor's Communication Handbook* – by Peter Tate, a leading GP consultation skills specialist.[54]

○ **Summary**

- Many patients now think and behave differently, and have varying expectations of professionals.

- Preparing GP registrars and others successfully for interacting with patients will have to involve the development of their capacities to deal with change and difference, and their ability to collaborate.

- Listening to learners and working with their needs are established principles in medical education, particularly communication learning.

- The process of doctors learning to do their own work of building on strengths to face change can help them to do the same for their patients.

- Work-based learning with a patient perspective can help professionals develop new approaches in clinical encounters with patients.

- There is no one right way to communicate; at the heart of the matter are questions of how we value others and think we can help them.

REFERENCES

1 Hart J T. *A New Kind of Doctor: The General Practitioner's Part in the Health of the Community.* London: Merlin Press, 1988.

2 Department of Health. *The Patient's Charter.* London: HMSO, 1991.

3 Department of Health. *Working for Patients.* London: HMSO, 1989.

4 Department of Health. *Building on the Best: Choice, Responsiveness and Equity in the NHS.* London: HMSO, 2003.

5 Wanless D. *Securing Our Future Health: Taking a Long-Term View.* London: HM Treasury, 2002.

6 *Challenges in Personal and Public Health Promotion.* Executive summary of conference of same title in 'Medicine for the 21st Century' series. Annenberg Centre. Eisenhower, Palm Springs, February 1992.

7 Kendall L and Lissauer R. *The Future Health Worker.* London: IPPR Publications, 2004.

8 Coulter A. Paternalism or partnership. *BMJ* 1999; **319**: 719–20.

9 Tuckett D, Boulton M, Olson C and Williams A. *Meetings with Experts. An Approach to Sharing Ideas in Medical Consultations.* London: Tavistock Publications, 1985.

10 Muir Gray J A. *The Resourceful Patient.* Oxford: eRosetta Press, 2002. Available as an 'e-book' and in print from www.resourcefulpatient.org [accessed August 2006].

11 Coulter A. *The Autonomous Patient: Ending Paternalism in Medical Care.* London: HMSO, 2002.

12 Launer J. *Narrative-Based Primary Care: A Practical Guide.* Oxford: Radcliffe Medical Press, 2002.

13 www.dipex.org [accessed August 2006].

14 Morris P, Burton K, Reiss M and Burton J. The difficult consultation. An action learning project about mental health issues in the consultation. *Education for General Practice* 2001; **12**: 19–26.

15 RCGP. Bromley-by-Bow Health Centre: holistic care in London's East End. *The New Generalist* 2004; **2**: 23–5.

16 Thistlethwaite J E, Green P D, Heywood P and Storr E. First step: report on a pilot course for personal and professional development. *Medical Education* 2000; **34**: 151–4.

17 Fitzpatrick M. Expert patients? *BJGP* 2004; **54**: 405.

18 Stewart M. Effective physician–patient communication and health outcomes: a review. *Canadian Medical Association Journal* 1995; **152**: 1423–33.

19 Salinsky J and Sackin P. *What Are You Feeling, Doctor? Identifying and Avoiding Defensive Patterns in the Consultation.* Oxford: Radcliffe Medical Press, 2000.

20 Dalton E and Griffiths J. Dealing with difficulties: overcoming emotional barriers to communication – a Cambridge experience. Invited plenary presentation at meeting at Royal Society of Medicine, 1998: Teaching Communication to Medical Undergraduates – Are We Advancing?

21 Burton J and Morris P. Mental illness or human distress? Challenges for primary care educators. *Education for General Practice* 2001; **12**: 1–10.

22 Campion P, Foulkes J, Neighbour R and Tate P. Patient-centredness in the MRCGP examination: analysis of large cohort. *BMJ* 2002; **325**: 691–2.

23 Blendon R J, Schoen C, Des Roches C, Osborn R and Zapert K. Common concerns amid diverse systems: health care experiences in five countries. *Health Affairs* 2003; **22**: 106–21.

24 Skelton J R. Everything you were afraid to ask about communication skills. *BJGP* 2005; **55**: 40–6.

25 Kidd J, Patel V, Peile E and Carter Y. Clinical and communication skills. *BMJ* 2005; **330**: 374–7.

26 Byrne P S and Long B E L. *Doctors Talking to Patients*. London: HMSO, 1967.

27 Bain D J G. Patient knowledge and the content of the consultation in general practice. *Medical Education* 1977; **11**: 347.

28 Willems S, De Maesschalck S, Deveugle M, Derese A and Maeseneer J. Socio-economic status of the patient and doctor–patient communication: does it make a difference? *Patient Education and Counseling* 2005; **56**: 139–46.

29 *Leadership for a Changing Profession*. London: MSD Foundation, 2002.

30 Whitehouse C, Morris P and Marks B. The role of actors in teaching medical communication. *Medical Education* 1984; **18**: 262–8.

31 Pendleton D, Schofield T, Tate P and Havelock P. *The Consultation: An Approach to Learning and Teaching*. Oxford: Oxford University Press, 1984.

32 Swaffield L. What is this bunch of actors doing in a hospital? *Nursing Times*, June 1982.

33 Pearson A, Morris P and Whitehouse C R. Consumer-orientated groups: a new approach to interdisciplinary teaching. *Journal of the Royal College of General Practitioners* 1985; **35**: 381–3.

34 Baker K. Dramatic changes. *BJGP* 2001; **51**: 598–9.

35 Morris P, Armitage A, Dalton E, Ewart B, Kilminster S, O'Neill F, *et al*. Patient involvement in learning about communication in healthcare: principles and methods. Workshop, European Association for Communication in Healthcare conference, Bruges, June 2005.

36 Baker K. Listening to women. Unpublished MPhil thesis. University of Sheffield, 2004.

37 Engels F. *The Condition of the Working Class in England in 1844*. London: Penguin, 1987 [originally published in 1845, this edition edited by VG Kiernan].

38 Freire P. *Pedagogy of the Oppressed*. Harmondsworth: Penguin, 1972.

39 Simpson M, Buckman R, Stewart M, *et al*. Doctor–patient communication: the Toronto consensus statement. *BMJ* 1991; **303**: 1385–7.

40 Lave J and Wenger E. *Situated Learning: Legitimate Peripheral Participation*. Cambridge: Cambridge University Press, 1991.

41 Maguire P, Fairbairn S and Fletcher C. Consultation skills of young doctors: I
    – benefits
    of feedback training in interviewing as students persist. *BMJ* 1986; **292**: 1573–8.

42 General Medical Council. *Recommendation on Basic Medical Education*. London: GMC,
    1980.

43 Wakeford R E. Communication skills training. In: Pendleton D and Hasler J (eds).
    Doctor Patient Communication. London: Academic Press, 1983, pp. 233–47.

44 Morris P. The development and evaluation of health education and information-
    giving skills for medical students and doctors. In: *Health Promotion: The Role of the
    Professional in the Community*. Cambridge: Health Promotion Research Trust, 1992,
    pp. 13–16.

45 Beckman H B and Frankel R M. The effect of physician behaviour on the collection of
    data. *Annals of Internal Medicine* 1984; **101**: 692–6.

46 Michie S, Miles J and Weinman J. Patient-centredness in chronic illness: what is it and
    what does it matter? *Patient Education and Counseling* 2004; **51**: 197–206.

47 Balint E, Courtenay M, Elder A, Hull S and Julian P. *The Doctor, the Patient and the
    Group: Balint Revisited*. London: Routledge, 1993.

48 Morris P, Dalton E, Griffiths J and Stanley M. Preparing for Patients: preparing
    tomorrow's doctors. *Patient Education and Counseling* 1998; **34**: S5–41.

49 Burton J and Launer J (eds). *Supervision and Support in Primary Care*. Oxford:
    Radcliffe, 2003.

50 West L. *Doctors on the Edge*. London: Free Association Books, 2001.

51 Rollnick S, Kinnersley P and Butler C. Context-bound communication skills training:
    development of a new method. *Medical Education* 2002; **36**: 377–83.

52 Wass V. Identifying and understanding the difficulties. Presented at 'Identifying and
    Supporting Medical Students with Communication Difficulties' meeting, 28 June
    2005. www.asme.org.uk/conf_courses/2005/06_28.htm [accessed October 2006].

53 Schofield T. A curriculum for communication in medical education. In: Macdonald E.
    (ed.) *Difficult Conversations in Medicine*. Oxford: Oxford University Press.

54 Tate P. *The Doctor's Communication Handbook*. Oxford: Radcliffe, 1994 (5th edition,
    2006).

Assessment of communication/ consultation skills and competence

What do we do and how do we do it?

This chapter explores issues relating to the assessment of skills and includes the following topics:

- competence versus performance • designing an assessment
- validity and reliability • the objective structured clinical examinations (OSCEs)
- the simulated surgery • videotaping of consultations • assessment by patients • portfolio-based assessment • communication/consultation rating scales/assessment instruments • the MRCGP examination of clinical competence • revalidation.

'For students preparing for Finals, the lottery of the sort of patient they may get for their 'long case' is a great source of worry. In general they hope for a patient with 'good' symptoms and signs ... but even more important is whether the patient is Co-operative or not ... students are told above all not to be rude to patients or to hurt them, and that this evidence that they are unfit to assume the Status of doctor is the only thing that may fail them outright.'

SIMON SINCLAIR, 1997

who carried out an ethnographic study of undergraduate medical education at University College London[1]

The assessment of clinical skills has been traditionally carried out by means of the long and short cases, both in medical finals and higher professional examinations. The membership examination of the Royal College of General Practitioners (RCGP) did not have a clinical skills-based component at all until 1995. Medical educators have challenged traditional case-based assessments on the grounds of subjectivity with regards to marking and lack of similarity to everyday practice. Current educational thinking is that to assess communication skills and interpersonal interactions, examination candidates should be observed interacting with patients. Assessments of videotaped consultations, simulated surgeries and OSCEs have been developed. The science behind the assessment of clinical skills, clinical competence and fitness to practise is being refined in order to improve the validity and reliability of such assessments. With revalidation now on the agenda for every doctor it is important to have valid and reliable ways of assessing consultation skills as one element of a doctor's professional competence.

The revalidation process has raised interest in methods for assessing performance. Demonstrating clinical competence is one of the more difficult aspects of this process. If assessment does drive learning[2] it would be hoped that ultimately regular assessment of clinical practice would improve consultation skills and thus outcomes for patients and possibly job satisfaction for doctors. However, this is by no means certain. As will be seen, doctors may change their usual behaviour when under scrutiny for assessment purposes. Unless this change in behaviour then persists in everyday practice the assessment will not improve standards.

There are a number of methods available for summative, formative, peer and self-assessment. There is a variety of people that may assess including GP trainers, tutors, peers, self and of course patients (real and simulated). All these will be considered in this chapter, which concentrates on more formal methods of assessment, rather than learning and feedback processes (covered in Chapters 5, 7 and 9).

Issues relating to assessment

Classical test theory is based on objective tests of knowledge rather than on performance-based assessments. In the last 30 years medical educators have concentrated their efforts on translating test theory to the latter though there are still many issues left to be discussed. In particular two important steps are not yet fully developed: methods of standard setting and clarification of the meaning of validity in performance assessment.[3]

○ **Competence** *the ability to do the job. What doctors do in controlled representations of professional practice.[4] Assessed in end-point examinations, usually under examination conditions.*

○ **Performance** *the ability to do the job well. What doctors do in their professional practice.[4] Assessed 'on the job' in clinical practice. Relates to continuing quality improvement.*

Assessment should ensure that a doctor is a competent medical practitioner. Qualifying examinations such as 'finals' and summative assessment following vocational training should prove that a doctor is competent at a defined level at that point in time. In terms of general practice this means that, having passed summative assessment, a doctor is competent to practise as an unsupervised general practitioner. Revalidation aims to show that a doctor remains competent. A single demonstration of competence, for example an assessment of one consultation, is not enough to prove adequate performance 'on the job' from day to day. There is a gap between competence and performance.[5]

Miller's pyramid[6] (Figure 8.1) represents a hierarchy of performance and is helpful in thinking about the kinds of assessment needed at different levels. A major priority in assessing competence of GPs is defining the depth and breadth of knowledge, and the appropriate skills and attitudes that *all* GPs should possess. This definition of competencies is made by professional and regulatory bodies. (GE Miller is a US psychologist.)

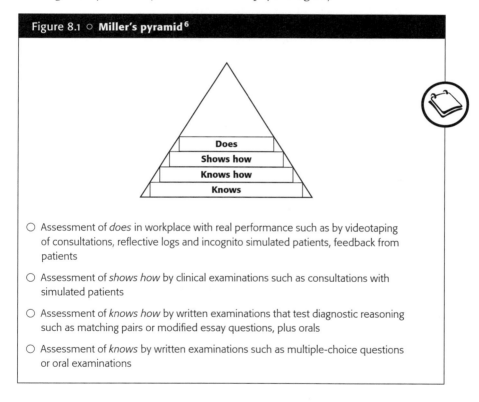

Figure 8.1 ○ Miller's pyramid[6]

- ○ Assessment of *does* in workplace with real performance such as by videotaping of consultations, reflective logs and incognito simulated patients, feedback from patients

- ○ Assessment of *shows how* by clinical examinations such as consultations with simulated patients

- ○ Assessment of *knows how* by written examinations that test diagnostic reasoning such as matching pairs or modified essay questions, plus orals

- ○ Assessment of *knows* by written examinations such as multiple-choice questions or oral examinations

A more difficult task is defining the elements of professional performance, as these differ depending on the situation in which a GP practises. A GP in a rural setting who provides intrapartum care needs a different set of knowledge and skills from a GP practising in an urban area with a high

Table 8.1 ○ **Components of performance**[7]

Component	Tasks
Clinical expertise	Patient diagnostic skills
	Patient management skills
Communication	With patients
	With colleagues
Collaboration	Teamwork
	Peer communication
Management	Personal management
	Systems management
	Clinical governance
	Resource utilisation
Personal development	Engaging in lifelong learning
	Developing insight into own limits
Education	Teaching students and junior doctors
	Helping patients understand their own health
	Research
	Critical appraisal
Professional attributes	Honesty
	Integrity
	Probity
	Respect for patients
	Respect for colleagues
	Ethical practice
Personal health and self-care	Self-care (mental, emotional, physical, spiritual)

concentration of non-English speaking patients, though there will be a great deal of overlap. A multinational group of medical educators has defined the components of performance that they feel should be assessed when ensuring a doctor remains fit to practise. Each component will vary in its details depending on the doctor's speciality and place of work. The list is interesting as many of the components can be thought of as directly relating to a consultation, and while one is identified as 'communication', communication skills are integral to most of the others. Therefore the list is given in full in Table 8.1.[7]

The RCGP has defined a syllabus for British general practice that is used as the basis of its current membership examination. This new curriculum for general practice training, which comes into force in August 2007, lists the knowledge, competencies, clinical and communication skills, and professional attributes considered necessary for unsupervised general practice.[8] Many of the items on this list are applicable to performance in consultations. The RCGP Curriculum Statement No.2 (see Chapter 1) outlines the core competencies related to the consultation.[9]

Designing an assessment

There are nine questions to consider when designing an assessment (Box 8.1). In reality, of course, there is no such thing as the 'ideal assessment'. Compromises have to be made in order for the assessment to be deliverable within a certain time and budget. The purpose of the assessment is of paramount importance. The purpose of summative assessment is well defined and well known to candidates. The purpose of a performance assessment is not always clear. Is it to identify poorly performing doctors? Is it to improve the standard of all candidates? Is it for regulatory purposes? The methods chosen will depend on the answers to these questions.

Box 8.1 ○ Designing an assessment

① What is the purpose of the assessment?

② Who is to be tested?

③ What competences are to be measured?

④ What is the blueprint for the assessment?

⑤ What method(s) should be used?

⑥ How are the scores to be defined?

⑦ What is the reliability of the assessment?

⑧ Is the assessment valid?

⑨ What are the standards against which the candidates are to be measured?

Traditionally the model of medical expertise used to design assessments considered the three domains of knowledge, skills and attitudes. A fourth domain of problem-solving skills was later added. In this model, communication and consultation behaviour are labelled as skills, thus needing a

---

Box 8.2 ○ **Validity and reliability**

Validity

How well a test or instrument measures what it should be measuring.

We would hope to be able to say: 'The higher the score, the better a doctor's consultation skills.'

Face validity

The instrument seems to either the assessors or developers to be measuring what it says it is measuring.

Criterion validity

The correlation of an instrument with other measures of the competence or attribute being assessed.

For example, comparing a GP registrar's score for a videotape consultation with an assessment by a patient and a trainer's report.

Reliability

The reproducibility or consistency of a test.

Inter-rater reliability

The ability of a test or instrument to produce similar results/scores when used by different observers.

'A doctor's score for a consultation should be similar when marked by two or more observers at the same time.'

Intra-rater reliability

The ability of a test or instrument to produce similar results/scores when used by the same observer on different days.

'A doctor's consultation should be scored the same if marked on different days by the same person.'

Inter-case (candidate) reliability

The ability of a test to measure consistency of a candidate performance across cases.

A candidate's marks should be broadly similar for each consultation in a simulated surgery.

---

skills-based assessment. However, the ideal consultation assessment will measure in all four domains, as these are all important during consultations. We tend to discuss consultation *skills*, often forgetting the important aspects of knowing what to do (knowledge) and the manner in which to do it (attitude), as well as how to do it (skill). The domains are not independent and more recently educationalists have been thinking in terms of roles or competences. For successful completion of a task or role, different aspects of medical competence have to be integrated.[10] The assessment blueprint (or detailed plan of the assessment structure) is the range of competences that are to be assessed across the whole examination and how this will be done. For example, explaining skills and knowledge relating to screening may be assessed by one OSCE station that involves the candidate explaining to a patient what a cervical smear is and how it is taken. The assessment blueprint ensures that each desired competence is covered in the examination at least once.

When designing an assessment tool for high-stakes examinations it is important to consider validity and reliability. As the terms are used frequently in medical education literature their definitions in relation to consultation skills are shown in Box 8.2.

Often validity is gained at the expense of reliability and vice versa. Intercase reliability is perhaps the most important issue in clinical competence testing,[11] as doctors do not perform consistently from consultation to consultation. A GP may be excellent at managing chronic disease and diagnosing rashes, but poor at involving patients in decisions and diagnosing depression. Confounding the issue still further one study has shown that doctors do not perform the same way with the same patient, with the same story, consulting six weeks apart (intra-doctor variation).[12] To make a valid judgement of a doctor's consultation competence, a large number of consultations involving a broad variety of clinical scenarios and patients should be observed and marked.

When assessment is used to judge whether a doctor reaches a certain standard, i.e. passes a certain mark, this pass mark must be set at the most fitting level. Setting the standard is usually done by criterion referencing and is decided before the assessment is marked. This is in contrast to peer referencing in which performance is described relative to the position of other candidates and only a pre-set number of candidates are allowed to pass the assessment. When carried out to the highest degree of accuracy, criterion referencing should involve setting standards for each element of an assessment, item by item. Thus the pass mark for a consultation skills assessment of competence involving several real or simulated consultations should not be the average of marks for each consultation. Rather each consultation should have an individual pass mark and the examiners should decide beforehand how many consultations should be passed in order to prove that a candidate has demonstrated competence.

Before considering 'what' should be assessed, we will discuss the various formats for 'how' this should be assessed. Other important features of an assessment when thinking of a format are its feasibility, i.e. whether it can be delivered within the constraints of resources and time; its acceptability to candidates, assessors, patients and society; and its educational impact, i.e.

the degree to which it helps candidates improve performance through preparation and feedback.[13] For high-stakes examinations legal defensibility is also important. As with most things in life, assessment formats come in and out of fashion. An example of this is the long case, which was discredited for a number of years. Student (candidate)/patient interaction was not observed and assessment was largely subjective in nature. However, certain educators are trying to rehabilitate the long case in the form of the OSLER (objective structured long examination record).[14] Within this format the examiners observe the candidate communicating and interacting with the patient. It is a 'long case' because history taking, examination and management are included. A structured marking sheet and extended marking scheme reduce the risk of subjectivity in marking.

Assessing 'shows how' by clinical examinations

To assess clinical competence with respect to communication and consultation skills some type of mock or simulated consultation scenario is set up.

The OSCE

A common format for the assessment of clinical skills is the OSCE. Since its development by Harden (of the Centre for Medical Education in Dundee) and Gleeson in 1979,[15] the OSCE has become a ubiquitous assessment, turning up in medical schools and some professional examinations (for example, the fellowship of the Royal Australian College of General Practitioners). The OSCE consists of a number of stations that help to give adequate sampling across various clinical scenarios and skills. Candidates rotate through the stations, which typically last from five to 10 minutes. The original concept was that all stations would include a 'patient' or clinical skill with a simulation (for example, 'taking blood' using a manikin) but stations often now include making sense of clinical data such as X-rays and blood results.

In terms of communication skills assessment the OSCE is a useful tool; however, it is limited by the length of the stations. Thus skills are often broken down into components. A station may be 'explaining' (explain to a patient what an endoscopy is), history taking (take a history from a patient with shortness of breath) or even breaking bad news (give the result of this abnormal chest X-ray to a patient). It is possible to have a long (or double) station but we would question the propriety of having only eight or even 16 minutes for such a complex task as breaking bad news. Of course given that the standard length of a British consultation is just under 10 minutes (9.36 minutes in 1997;[16] 9.4 minutes in 2004[17]), it should be possible to assess the complexity of the skills involved in consultations in a 10-minute station. However, doctor–patient interactions in GP consultations are rarely one-off situations, as the patient's ongoing story is often well known. Moreover, doctors will allow consultations to run over time if necessary and they have the potential to see the patient again as appropriate.

Assessment of communication and attitudes is made more difficult by the finding that these attributes are case specific.[10] Excellent performance with one patient may be followed by poor performance with another. A doctor's level of competence is not generalisable across such stations. To assess empathy, for instance, as many as 37 different cases would be needed.[18]

As with any 'new' assessment tool, the OSCE has been subjected to much stringent evaluation over the years. One criticism of the format is that examinees may do well on a checklist of items, for example asking about a patient's concerns, without fully understanding or engaging with the process.[19] Another criticism is that assessment instruments shape professional behaviour. Thus the OSCE defines and reinforces particular behaviour among candidates both before, and for some time after, they take the examination because its content sends out a message about what is considered important in medical practice.[20] This is not necessarily a bad thing if candidates deduce that sharing understanding and decisions with patients is important, and they do not only behave in this way in examinations. However, to know this we would have to see if such behaviour was reproduced a long while after the assessment and in the workplace.

The RCGP will introduce an OSCE-type examination as its clinical examination from 2007. It will build on the experience as an assessment tool.

The simulated surgery

An OSCE is only valid if it reproduces as far as possible the authentic clinical situation in which the candidates have to produce competent behaviours. Lack of authenticity occurs even in regards to such a simple fact that OSCE candidates rotate round the stations, whereas in practice the patients would come to them. To improve authenticity the simulated surgery has been developed. In 1997 the simulated surgery was introduced as an alternative method of assessment to videotaping real surgeries for the consultation skills element of the MRCGP examination. The blueprint for the consultation skills assessment includes all the relevant components of a general practice consultation – problem-solving skills, clinical management, personal care, oral communication and the consultation process – and these are covered in the simulated surgery.

The format of the surgery differs slightly in the two assessments for which it has been used: the MRCGP examination and summative assessment. It consists of eight to 12 cases lasting up to 10 minutes each. The doctor sits in the consulting room and the patients rotate round the rooms. For the membership examination a medical observer accompanies the patient and marks the candidate in the domains of information gathering, doctor–patient interaction (including awareness of the patient's concerns), communication and explanation, management, and anticipatory care.

For summative assessment only the patient marks and no examiner is necessary. The cases are worked up from videotapes of real patient consultations. There are two marking sheets. One focuses on the diagnostic and management aspects of the consultation (content, see below) and one on the communication skills and doctor–patient interaction/rapport (process). The first sheet is a series of items that are specific to the case, for example if a patient complains of rectal bleeding the candidate would be marked on whether they asked about family history. Though the simulated patient (SP) marks each sheet, the content sheet is objective in that the patient does not know the relative weighting of each item and is only marking on the basis on what the doctor says or does. The communication sheet is more subjective and is based on what the patient (in role) feels about the doctor's performance in relation to rapport building, explaining skills and involving the patient in management decisions. Physical examination skills are not tested.[21]

Candidates who have taken this assessment have commented on its validity, though it has some limitations in that no consultations involve children, emergency cases, physical signs or are with patients previously known to the doctor.[22] Cases should be chosen to cover the whole spectrum of general practice, with patients with a spread of ages and both genders, with acute and chronic problems, common and less common conditions, and health promotion activities. Pass marks are assigned to each individual consultation and candidates have to pass a minimum number of consultations to pass the whole assessment.

Currently the College will only allow candidates to sit simulated surgeries in place of the video assessment of clinical skills (see below) in cases of 'insuperable' difficulties in obtaining a video recording. These might for example include the candidate practising in an area where few people speak English, where it might be difficult to obtain consent from patients and if the candidate is not working regularly in the same practice.

Assessing 'does' by clinical examinations

Ultimately the most valid assessment of consultation skills and clinical per-

---

Box 8.3 ○ Methods of assessing 'does'

○ Rating of videotapes of consultations.

○ Medical observer sits in with the doctor on consultations.

○ Incognito (covert) SP assesses doctor.

○ Asking patients for feedback on a doctor's performance.

○ Reflective portfolios.

○ Multi-source assessment including 360 degree appraisal.

---

formance is by testing what the doctor does from day to day in the workplace: in the surgery and in the home. This is an assessment of 'does', the doctor's actual performance. There are six main ways in which 'does' may be assessed, all of which have advantages and disadvantages (Box 8.3). For the assessment of performance ideally evidence should be collected by means of a combination of these instruments, but this reduces the feasibility and acceptability while increasing the cost. However, content specificity, measuring clinical performance across a broad range of doctor–patient interactions and by these different means, is crucial for the assessment of professional performance within consultations.

Videotaping consultations

This method of assessment has been used for both summative assessment at the end of general practice vocational training to decide on fitness to practise as an unsupervised GP and in the membership examination of the RCGP.* The assessment method has a high degree of validity and reliability. However, GP trainers report that registrars spend an inordinate amount of time selecting and editing consultations in order to give a good impression and gain high marks. Yet reflection on why a consultation went 'badly' in the opinion of the doctor is also a sign of consultation maturity. A criticism that we have of this method is that the patient voice is not heard. The examining doctors decide on whether the candidate has explained the diagnosis and management plan to the patient and whether management decisions have been shared with the patient. However, from watching a tape one cannot really judge whether the patient has understood the explanation or felt involved.

For the RCGP examination candidates must provide a tape of seven consultations and write a commentary on each one. As well as giving brief details about the case, the commentary must include 50 words reflecting on the setting of the consultation, what was achieved and what issues may arise later. The recordings submitted for summative assessment must be of

---

*NOTE With effect from 3 February 2007, all those wishing to apply to sit the membership examination of the RCGP will be required to complete the new assessment package (nMRCGP).

two hours' duration and comprise no fewer than eight consultations. The single route to both MRCGP and summative assessment allows submission of one videotape fulfilling these requirements.[23]

Consideration must be given to issues of patient consent to be taped. There are standard consent forms for assessment purposes. Patients may be reluctant to be taped if they want to discuss very personal or embarrassing problems. Some patients do not want to be taped on religious or cultural grounds. This reduces the mix of patients and therefore the validity to some extent. Intimate physical examinations will not be recorded either. However, overall this method gives a good perspective of a doctor's performance, and doctors who have been assessed by this method say they recognise their usual daily performance in the videotaped consultations.[24]

Medical observer sits in on consultations

This method is more likely to be used for formative assessment, though it does have high face validity. As feedback may be given immediately it is useful as a learning experience. The observer may also be able to watch examination technique. Technical problems include the patient not fully understanding the role of the observer, the patient directing remarks to both doctors and the observed doctor being understandably nervous, which may affect performance. Doctors may also alter their normal behaviour when being observed, but at least this suggests that they know what behaviour is considered to be acceptable.

Incognito SPs

In the UK the use of SPs to study the performance of GPs has been mainly overt (the doctor knows that the patients are simulators) rather than covert (when the doctor is unaware of this fact[25]). In the Netherlands,[26] New Zealand[27] and Canada,[28] SPs have been used posing as 'real' patients for the validation or assessment of GPs' performance and also in secondary care settings.[29] The use of SPs in this way has been shown to be a valid method for assessing actual clinical performance in the workplace.[30]

The rationale is that if the doctors are unaware that the patient is a simulator, their clinical performance is likely to be more authentic and not simply a test of competence. However, there are logistical problems to overcome when trying to introduce a SP into a general practice surgery without the doctor knowing.[31] Before introducing incognito patients into a clinical setting, GPs should be familiar with the use of overt SPs. This is likely to be the case with doctors who are recently qualified, as the use of SPs is well established in medical schools and is becoming so on vocational training schemes. Moreover, as previously discussed a full assessment of competence cannot be made on the basis of one consultation, so this method would have to be combined with others.

The use of SPs in this manner does raise ethical issues.[32] Before introducing the method as a formal assessment of competence such issues should be addressed. Practice staff need to be fully informed of what is happening and why. Special care needs to be paid to the scenario and status of the SP. To account for the fact that the patient has very few notes, if any, the SP will normally be acting as a temporary resident or new patient, which may affect the way the consultation is conducted. Ideally SPs should be involved in developing the scenario, particularly if there is the potential that a physical examination is likely given the patient's history. However, consultations of this type are best used to assess a doctor's communication skills rather than examination. The scenario should ideally be based on the case of a real patient. As soon as possible after the consultation the doctor should be informed of the identity of the SP to reduce ensuing problems relating to further management or anxiety. The marking sheet is obviously important, as is the decision as to what exactly the patient is assessing.

Asking patients for feedback

This may be done directly after a consultation or later by interview or questionnaire. Patients are only able to assess in certain domains and this method should be combined with others to gain a complete picture of the doctor's consultation skills and knowledge. It is an indirect measure of performance and relies on the memory of a patient who will have concerns other than assessing the doctor. Competence cannot be directly correlated with patient satisfaction,[33] as doctors may legitimately decline to behave inappropriately, to the dissatisfaction of the patient, for example in the case of filling out insurance forms with incorrect details. Thus validity and reliability are poor. However, such dissatisfaction often has its root in poor communication.

Issues relating to assessment by patients

Both real and simulated patients are being asked to make judgements about patients. Certainly in training sessions SPs are a valuable source of formative feedback. For summative assessment SPs must be consistent in their role-play,[34] which is why they are sometimes referred to as standardised patients. The evidence suggests that doctors' competence can be assessed reliably by SPs.[27,35] Real patients are obviously less reliable but they have a valuable contribution to make in the assessment of doctors' interpersonal and communication skills. Only patients can really say if they have understood what the doctor has told them, if they felt involved in decision making and if their views were valued. A medical observer cannot really know this.

Thus the patient voice should be canvassed at some time in the assessment process.

Patients cannot assess medical knowledge, though some are provided with checklists written by professionals to try to do this. As not all doctors think or work in the same way such checklists may not capture the true essence of a doctor's performance. Some doctors may not need to cover all the items on a checklist to reach the same conclusion about diagnosis and management. A patient could not know this and may penalise some doctors unfairly. Patients are now being involved in devising the checklists to validate them further. A major contribution that patients have, particularly in formative assessment, is the impact of their feedback on doctors' skill development:[36] the patient voice is a powerful tool, as we describe further in Chapter 9.

Portfolios

○ **Portfolio** *a purposeful collection of work intended to demonstrate a person's ability within a particular field. In the education/assessment sense usually includes evidence that learning has taken place.*

Portfolios are increasingly being recognised as a means of helping doctors in their continuing professional development as well as undergraduate and postgraduate education. They usually include documentation of learning and a reflective account of those documented events.[37] At first sight a portfolio would seem to be a poor method for the assessment of consultation skills. However, in conjunction with other methods it can be useful. Portfolios could include a consultation diary, with lists of patients and conditions, to provide evidence that a GP, GP registrar or student has seen a wide range of presentations in patients of all ages and circumstances. The portfolio could also include measures of patient satisfaction with the consultations, outcome data (what happened next) and peer assessment of consultations through analysis of videotapes or sitting in.

The problem is with the reflective element. Portfolios may become simple repositories of data collection. Reflection helps show that the doctor has learned from the consultation, has thought about their skills, evaluated them and used the evaluation to plan changes to improve skills or knowledge. The challenge then is to be able to assess this reflection. The reliability of any such assessment will be low. Reflection is considered in more detail in Chapter 7.

The UK revalidation of doctors, a process giving them the right to continue to practise, will almost certainly involve doctors keeping a folder of evidence (or portfolio) of what they have been doing in the past five years. As well as including elements relating to communication skills, such evidence could also comprise prescribing data, audits and some form of multi-source assessment.[38]

Multi-source assessment

Also called 360 degree assessment or feedback,[39] this is a combination of methods by different assessors, including patients, peers, practice staff and other health professionals, looking at the same doctor. This increases the criterion validity, but has major resource and financial implications. This method is probably the only one that can look at how well a GP works within a team. Team-working is a hallmark of modern primary care and needs good communication skills but it is rarely assessed.[40] At present there is limited evidence confirming the reliability and validity of this method, and the role of patients and peers within such an assessment system.[41]

Rating the consultation

So far we have explored the methods of assessing consultations and communication skills, attempting to answer the question 'How do we measure such skills?' But we also need to consider the questions 'What do we measure?' and 'How do we score a consultation?' Underlying these questions are two more difficult ones, 'What are the hallmarks of good consultation skills?' and 'How do we know if a GP is competent at consulting?' As consultations are very complex interactions, any valid and reliable assessment must measure knowledge and attitude as well as skills.

All of the methods of assessment for 'shows how' and 'does' described above need to be combined with some sort of marking /assessment instrument or rating scale in order to determine the doctor's competence and/or performance. The scale may be completed by the patient (real or simulated), a medically trained observer or assessor (usually senior to the candidate) or by a peer for revalidation purposes. Rating scales vary not only in content but also in the method or marking. Some have Likert scales, while some have defined parameters, and some have space to write in comments and some grade simply as pass/fail.

There are a large number of scales and assessment instruments for assessing consultation skills in the literature. The items on these scales are usually chosen by canvassing the opinion of groups of doctors, including academics, on what should happen in a consultation. Medical schools and GP training programmes develop rating scales for use locally for either teaching and/or assessment, but often do not publish their experiences of such use. Those that are published have usually been evaluated for validity and reliability to some extent. Some scales focus on content and some on process as discussed below (and also see Chapter 2). Some try to combine both elements. There are instruments that focus on specific aspects of the consultation, such as its patient-centredness or the extent to which shared decision making is taking place.

When searching for a suitable instrument, attention must be paid to whether it was devised for use in teaching, formative or summative assessment. Scales and instruments to help learning and skill development are not usually subjected to rigorous testing for validity and reliability. However, when considering summative assessment tools it is salutary to read a paper by Evans (a clinical research fellow) and colleagues from the University of Wales. They performed a systematic literature review in 2004 to identify instruments for the peer assessment of doctors, in particular instruments that assess the humanistic aspects of doctor–patient interactions such as integrity, empathy and consultation skills.[42] Of the many instruments described they only found three (two from the USA and one from Canada) that fitted their criterion of having psychometric data about their validity established. None of the reviewed instruments, including these three, had a theoretical framework. The two US instruments had only been used in hospitals. The Canadian one, the peer assessment questionnaire, is based on a grid of competences including communication and psychosocial management derived from a professional committee.[43]

Three years earlier, in 2001, some of the same team from Wales had carried out a similar systematic review but this time looking for instruments that measured the involvement of patients in shared decision making specifically. They found that little attention had been given to assessing patient involvement except as a minor component of other competences.[44] Moreover, in a small study of their own they found little correlation between scores for patient-centredness and shared decision making, leading to the conclusion that patient-centred communication and shared decision making are conceptually different, particularly in relation to current definitions.[45] This led them to develop their own scale (the OPTION – observing patient involvement – instrument), which is discussed later in the chapter.

Mead and Bower of the National Primary Care Research Centre in Manchester evaluated approaches to measuring the patient-centredness of consultations based on their own model of the concept derived from the literature.[46] They argued that the 'development of valid and reliable measures is constrained by lack of theoretical clarity and the inevitable difficulties of measuring complex processes'.

In the following sections we describe some assessment instruments and rating scales, how and when they may be used, and their limitations. Questions still remain about the validity of trying to assess such criteria as empathy, respect and integrity. Moreover, detailed checklists have been shown not to be as objective as originally thought.[47] Global marking, which is when an examiner gives an overall mark based on the totality of the performance, has been shown to be as reliable as checklists as long as the examiners receive adequate training.[48] However, checklists are useful for giving candidates feedback, if this is built into the assessment procedure, or for providing proof of what happened in the assessment if a candidate contests their marks. Checklists also drive behaviour, as they show examinees what is expected of them. However, as mentioned above, behaviour does not always reflect understanding of the process; examinees may learn such behaviours 'parrot fashion' without engaging fully with the patient.

Content and process

A simple way of breaking down the consultation for assessment purposes is into content and process (Box 8.4). Knowledge, skills and attitudes are components of both content and process.

Box 8.4 ○ Content and process

Content

○ What happens.

○ The quality of the information gathered and shared.

○ The diagnosis.

○ Knowledge of the medical condition.

○ The management plan.

○ Advice about risk factors and disease prevention.

Process (behaviour)

○ How it happens.

○ Communication skills.

○ Shared decision-making skills.

○ Patient-centred approach.

In some situations the assessor may wish to concentrate on content and discuss medical knowledge and its application, the results of investigations and the choice of management. In other cases the assessor may wish to con-

---

Box 8.5 ○ **The MRCGP elements of clinical competence**

Tasks

1. Discover the reason for the patient's attendance.
2. Define the clinical problems(s).
3. Explain the problem(s) to the patient.
4. Address the patient(s)' problems.
5. Make effective use of the consultation.

Performance criteria

1. The doctor is seen to encourage the patient's contribution at appropriate points in the consultation.
2. The doctor is seen to respond to signals (cues) that lead to a deeper understanding of the problem (M).
3. The doctor uses appropriate psychological and social information to place the complaint(s) in context.
4. The doctor explores the patient's health understanding.
5. The doctor obtains sufficient information to include or exclude likely relevant significant conditions.
6. The physical/mental examination chosen which is likely to confirm or disprove hypotheses that could reasonably have been formed OR is designed to address a patient's concern.
7. The doctor appears to make a clinically appropriate working diagnosis.
8. The doctor explains the diagnosis in appropriate language.
9. The doctor's explanation incorporates some or all of the patient's health beliefs (M).
10. The doctor specifically seeks to confirm the patient's understanding of the diagnosis (M).
11. The management plan (including any prescription) is appropriate for the working diagnosis, reflecting a good understanding of modern accepted medical practice.
12. The patient is given the opportunity to be involved in significant management decisions.
13. The doctor takes steps to enhance concordance, by exploring and responding to the patient's understanding of the treatment (M).
14. The doctor specifies the appropriate conditions and interval for follow-up or review.

centrate on content including rapport building, diagnostic reasoning and how the patient was involved in decision making. In most situations the assessor will want to look at both content and process.

The MRCGP statement of clinical competence

The current membership examination for the RCGP is the best-developed assessment in the UK. Clinical competence was defined by a working group in 1990[49] and was derived from the task model of Pendleton and colleagues.[50] The criteria for competence are divided into units (tasks), elements (strategies) and performance criteria (skills). The tasks are broken down into the elements. Each element has one or more performance criteria, a total of 14, of which four attract a merit (M) mark. It is these criteria that may be more reliably assessed (Box 8.5).[51]

Criteria 1, 2, 4, 9, 10, 12 and 13 are those that reflect the patient-centredness of a consultation. It is interesting to look at the results of the MRCGP examination as a measure of what doctors are doing in consultations. As the above criteria were modified in 2004 and their numbering was changed, the results cannot be directly related to the list above. However, the previously defined criteria involving the doctor taking the patient's health understanding into account, utilising the patient's health beliefs during explaining and confirming the patient's understanding were not seen in 14 per cent, 31 per cent and 45 per cent of doctors' submitted tapes respectively. Involving patients in decision making was also rare, with only 36 per cent of doctors demonstrating this in their first five consultations.[52] In the 2002 diet of examinations, a quarter of candidates for both summative assessment and the membership examination failed solely for not showing sufficient evidence of involving patients in shared decision making.[53] Given that we must assume that most doctors submit their best consultations for scrutiny, this is a worrying finding, raising questions about training in consultation skills. However, some candidates try to play safe and submit too many consultations for minor illness and repeat prescriptions, where shared decision making may not be relevant. (A new format for the MRCGP will be introduced in 2007.)

The northern trainers' instrument for the assessment of videotapes of GPs' consultations

This instrument, described by GPs Cox and Mulholland in 1993, was developed by asking GP trainers, GP registrars, experienced GPs and patients in the north of England what were the important characteristics of a competent GP. The rating scale that resulted has 37 statement pairs separated by a six-point scale. Assessors are asked to mark on the scale at a point that most closely agrees with their assessment of the candidate's performance. For example, two statements are: the patient is not involved in decision making – the patient is involved in decision making.[54]

The complexity of this scale means that it is hard to use when observing consultations other than by videotaping, as it is difficult to observe performance and mark at the same time. Videotaping allows replaying of chunks of the consultation to check scoring. The statements are not really in a logical order in our opinion, but it is a useful instrument for discussion of consultation skills. Some of the statements would be best scored by the patient, for example 'the patient understands the doctor' and 'the doctor allows time for the patient'.

The Leicester assessment package (LAP)

This assessment of consultation competences was developed mainly by Robin Fraser, Professor of General Practice at Leicester University, from work undertaken in Leicester and Kuwait. It can be used in real and simulated settings. It consists of seven categories of competences, with 39 components. It includes both behavioural and professional components unlike the Cox and Mulholland instrument, which only includes the former. Of relevance to communication are: interviewing/history taking; patient management (e.g. formulates management plans – in collaboration with patients); behaviour/relationship with patients. The package comes with observer recording forms, criteria for the allocation of scores and questions that assessors may ask during consultations to probe the doctor's reasoning. The face validity was checked by a questionnaire survey of British course organisers.[55] The LAP has been shown to have high reliability for the assessment of British GPs[56] and is used for the assessment of competence around the world, for example in New Zealand, Hong Kong and Hungary.

A pilot study of volunteer GPs who agreed to be assessed using the LAP proved to be a positive experience for these 24 experienced doctors. The GPs welcomed the opportunity to affirm their competence while recognising the need to improve their skills as a continual process.[57] However, as a voluntary (formative) assessment and without the real power of revalidation it would be hoped that the experience was useful. Summative assessment for revalidation would be a much more anxiety-provoking process.

The OPTION (observing patient involvement) instrument

This instrument was developed by a team from the University of Wales and was based on data collected from 186 audiotaped consultations of 21 GPs. It aims to assess the extent to which doctors involve patients in the decision-making process. There are full psychometric data for its reliability and valid-

---

Box 8.6 ○ The OPTION instrument[59]

① Identification of problem(s) needing a decision-making process.

② Equipoise statements (see Chapter 3).

③ Listing options, including 'no action'.

④ Explaining options.

⑤ Information format, e.g. words, numbers, visual display.

⑥ Exploring expectations.

⑦ Exploring concerns.

⑧ Checking understanding.

⑨ Opportunities for questions.

⑩ Eliciting the patient's preferred level of involvement.

⑪ Making (or deferring) a decision.

⑫ Reviewing the decision (follow-up).

---

ity.[58] When used to grade GPs it shows, as might be expected, that individuals vary from consultation to consultation in the amount to which they do involve patients. This may reflect the flexibility of some in responding to the nature of the patient's problem or the patient's preference for wishing to be involved. Overall GPs who were assessed with the instrument scored low marks, suggesting that further skills development is needed in this area, a finding that matches those of the MRCGP examiners discussed above. The 12 items of OPTION are listed in Box 8.6. The first is a 'gateway' item; obviously the rest of the instrument cannot be used if this first item is not achieved.

The patient enablement instrument (PEI)

This instrument was developed in Edinburgh as a means for patients to assess the quality of a general practice consultation (Table 8.2). The assessment is based on the assumption that how a patient feels after a consultation is an important factor in predicting outcome.[60] The PEI is a measure of patient satisfaction and may be used as one piece of evidence in a portfolio to demonstrate performance. It also pays attention to the notion that the purpose of the consultation is to support patients to manage themselves better; it can thus act as a 'driver' for patient involvement in the consultation. The enablement score is likely to be higher if the patient knows the doctor well[61] and thus this is not an instrument for assessment in a simulated scenario.

There are many more instruments for the measurement of patient satisfaction in the literature. It is worth noting that patient satisfaction is relative to patient expectation. Patients who do not expect a high level of care will have their expectations easily met. Therefore the positive ratings of their experience may not necessarily reflect higher standards of care. Patient satisfaction is context specific and is not simply a matter of analysing the results from validated questionnaires unless a prior assessment of patient expectation has been made.[62]

Table 8.2 ○ **PEI**[60]

As a result of your visit to the doctor today do you feel you are	Much better	Better	Same or less	N/A
able to cope with life?				
able to understand your illness?				
able to cope with your illness?				
able to keep yourself healthy?				
	Much more	More	Same or less	N/A
confident about your health?				
able to help yourself?				

Issues relating to revalidation

Revalidation has been mentioned several times in this chapter as the process involves assessment of clinical competence. The General Medical Council (GMC) will introduce periodic revalidation for all doctors on the medical register in 2007; the official format this will take is still under discussion.[63] In order to retain a licence to practise doctors have to show that they remain up to date and competent every five years. They do this by producing verifiable evidence from their day-to-day medical practice that is appropriate to their speciality and type of practice. Revalidation must include regular reflection on performance and participation in the annual appraisal scheme.

Doctors must provide evidence to show that they conform to the requirements of good medical practice as defined by the GMC.[64] Criteria for acceptable practice include the communication and consultation skills already defined in this book. Due to problems with feasibility and resource implications doctors provide evidence of these skills by confirmation by peers and/or patients. This may change once revalidation is embedded in professional life. Doctors who cause concern are assessed by a more robust clinical examination. However, as we have already discussed there are problems relating to all types of clinical assessment of competence or performance.

Assessment ○ *reflections*

My generation of medical students had to pass finals: a written and clinical examination in each speciality followed by a viva. There was no general practice assessment. The clinical examinations were long and short cases. At no stage was I observed interacting with a patient during the history-taking phase of a case. For MRCGP there were also written papers and a long viva. Patients were noticeably absent from the examination. Of course, this has all changed. Observation of clinical and communication skills is now standard practice in assessments, though there is still disagreement about marking sheets and the role of the patient's perspective. So how would I like to be assessed for revalidation? Only on the job please. I have no objections to incognito SPs and I am well used to being videotaped, but I have found an observer sitting in a distraction to both the patient and myself. However, I feel that a variety of evidence is needed and that it should be my responsibility to provide the type of evidence that demonstrates my competence and my performance. This evidence will depend on where I work, the type of practice, my special skills and other work. It sounds like a portfolio to me.

As a profession we should expect to provide evidence that our practice meets acceptable performance standards. Patients have the right to know that their doctors meet such standards. The main questions are what should be the standards, who sets them and how are they measured. The 360 degree appraisal system would include patients' views but would need to involve patient training to carry out such assessment.

Assessment and feedback ○ *reflections*

Wherever I work, people do seem to know when someone hasn't communicated well. During examinations or on the job, be it in OSCEs, on a ward, in a general practice, colleagues and patients can spot this, i.e. they can assess a core clinical skill very effectively. So what is the problem with making sure that this is addressed for the sake of patients' safety? Well, sometimes it's hard to feed back, especially for patients who don't want to risk not being taken care of. And then it's hard to keep track of feedback. For example, some years ago, one medical student was finally identified at a third-year OSCE as someone who really struggled, for many reasons, to communicate at all and who therefore could not function clinically. So how had we missed him? Partly, we hadn't – there was a report from his communication skills tutor in his first year, worrying about his communication in his group. That had just remained on file. In the second year, simulated patients had complained about him, but we did not count their feedback then. Then ward reports where nurses and doctors all had to mark 'communication skills' either had a mark in the middle of the scale, or no mark. Clinically, he had just got by in groups, somehow, hiding his difficulties. He had been given little feedback. This sort of thing still happens with trainees and practitioners, and will do more often, as doctors move about more. People feel sorry for those in difficulty, few trust that feedback will be heard or feel confident that anything can be done to help, everyone hopes someone else will take it up, so it's all smudged, not faced. It will help if individual feedback becomes the norm, with reliable tracking systems and clear opportunities for improvement available to all, so it's not stigmatising to get help.

○ Summary

- Assessment should ensure that a doctor is a competent medical practitioner.

- Revalidation aims to show that a doctor remains competent.

- A major priority in assessing competence of GPs is defining the depth and breadth of knowledge, and the appropriate skills and attitudes that all GPs should possess.

- When designing an assessment tool for high-stakes examinations it is important to consider validity and reliability.

- Inter-case reliability is perhaps the most important issue in clinical competence testing, as doctors do not perform consistently from consultation to consultation.

- The development of valid and reliable measures for assessing clinical competence is difficult as consultations are complex interactions.

- Patients should be involved in the assessment of doctors but consideration needs to be given to what they can assess reliably.

- There are many instruments and rating scales for assessing consultation skills but few have been adequately evaluated or have theoretical underpinning.

REFERENCES

1 Sinclair S. *Making Doctors. An Institutional Apprenticeship.* Oxford: Berg, 1997. p. 241.

2 Newble D and Jaeger K. The effects of assessment and examinations on the learning of medical students. *Medical Education* 1983; **17**: 165–71.

3 Ben-David M F. Life beyond OSCE. *Medical Teacher* 2003; **25**: 239–40.

4 Rethans J-J, Norcini J J, Baron-Maldonado M, *et al.* The relationship between competence and performance: implications for assessing practice performance. *Medical Education* 2002; **36**: 901–9.

5 Rethans J-J, Sturmans F, Drop R, van der Vleuten C and Hobus P. Does competence of general practitioners predict their performance? Comparison between examination setting and actual practice. *BMJ* 1991; **303**: 1377–80.

6 Miller G E. The assessment of clinical skills/competence/performance. *Academic Medicine* (Supplement) 1990; **65**: S63–7.

7 Hays R B, Davies H A, Beard J D, *et al.* Selecting performance assessment methods for experienced physicians. *Medical Education* 2002; **36**: 910–17.

8 Look for examinations information on: www.rcgp.org.uk.

9 Look for examinations information on: www.rcgp.org.uk.

10 Schuwirth L W T and van der Vleuten C. Changing education, changing assessment, changing research? *Medical Education* 2004; **38**: 805–12.

11 Wass V, van der Vleuten C, Shatzer J and Jones R. Assessment of clinical competence. *Lancet* 2001; **357**: 945–9.

12 Rethans J J and Saebu L. Do general practitioners act consistently in real practice when they meet the same patient twice? Examination of intradoctor variation using standardized (simulated) patients. *BMJ* 1997; **314**: 1170.

13 Van der Vleuten C. The assessment of professional competence: developments, research and practical implications. *Advances in Health Sciences Education* 1996; **1**: 41–67.

14 Gleeson F. Assessment of clinical competence using the objective structured long examination record (OSLER). *Medical Teacher* 1997; **19**: 7–14.

15 Harden R A and Gleeson F A. ASME medical educational booklet No 8: assessment of medical competence using an objective structured clinical examination (OSCE). *Journal of Medical Education* 1979; **13**: 41–54.

16 RCGP. *General Practice Workload. Information Sheet No 3*. London: RCGP, 2004.

17 Deveugle M, Derese A, Brink-Muinen A, Bensing J and de Maeseneer J. Consultation length in general practice: cross sectional study in six European countries. *BMJ* 2002; **325**: 472.

18 Colliver J A, Willis M S, Robbs R S, Cohen D S and Swartz M H. Assessment of empathy in a standardized patient examination. *Teaching and Learning in Medicine* 1998; **10**: 8–11.

19 Wass V and Jolly B. Does observation add to the validity of the long case? *Medical Education* 2001; **35**: 729–34.

20 Hodges B. Validity and the OSCE. *Medical Teacher* 2003; **25**: 250–4.

21 Allen J, Evans A, Foulkes J and French A. Simulated surgery in the summative assessment of general practice training: results of a trial in the Trent and Yorkshire regions. *BJGP* 1998; **48**: 1219–23.

22 Burrows P J and Bingham L. The simulated surgery – an alternative to videotape submission for the consulting skills element of the MRCGP examination: the first year's experience. *BJGP* 1999; **49**: 269–72.

23 www.rcgp.org.uk/exams/examination_home/examination_information/video_workbook.aspx [accessed September 2006].

24 Ram P, Grol R, Rethans J-J, Schouten B, van der Vleuten C and Kester A. Assessment of general practitioners by video observation of communicative and medical performance in daily practice: issues of validity, reliability and feasibility. *Medical Education* 1999; **33**: 447–54.

25 Kinnersley P and Pill R. Potential of using simulated patients to study the performance of general practitioners. *BJGP* 1993; **43**: 297–9.

26 Rethans J-J, Sturmans F, Drop R and van der Vleuten C. Assessment of the performance of general practitioners by the use of standardized (simulated) patients. *BJGP* 1991; **41**: 97–9.

27 O'Hagan J J, Davies L J and Pears R K. The use of simulated patients in the assessment of actual clinical performance in general practice. *New Zealand Medical Journal* 1986; **99**: 948–51.

28 Renaud M, Beauchemin J, Lalonde C, *et al.* Practice settings and prescribing profiles: the simulation of tension headaches to general practitioners working in different practice settings in the Montreal area. *American Journal of Public Health* 1990; **70**: 1068–73.

29 Gorter S L, Rethans J-J, Scherpier A J J A, *et al.* How to introduce incognito standardized patients into outpatient clinics of specialists in rheumatology. *Medical Teacher* 2001; **23**: 138–44.

30 Van der Vleuten C and Swanson D. Assessment of clinical skills with standardized patients: state of the art. *Teaching and Learning in Medicine* 1990; **2**: 58–76.

31 Thistlethwaite J E. The use of incognito simulated patients in general practice: a feasibility study. *Education for Primary Care* 2003; **14**: 419–25.

32 Neighbour R. Reflections on the ethics of assessment. *Education for Primary Care* 2003; **14**: 406–10.

33 Baker R. Pragmatic model of patient satisfaction in general practice: progress towards a theory. *Quality Health Care* 1997; **6**: 201–4.

34 Barrows H S. An overview of the uses of standardized patients for teaching and evaluating clinical skills. *Academic Medicine* 1993; **68**: 443–51.

35 Vu N V, Barrows H, Marcy M, Verhulst S J, Colliver J A and Travis T. Six years of comprehensive clinical performance based assessment using standardised patients at the Southern Illinois University School of Medicine. *Academic Medicine* 1992; **62**: 42–50.

36 Greco M, Brownlea A and McGovern J. Impact of patient feedback on interpersonal skills of general practice registrars: results of a longitudinal study. *Medical Education* 2001; **35**: 748–56.

37 Snadden D and Thomas M L. The use of portfolio learning in medical education. *Medical Teacher* 1998; **20**: 192–9.

38 Esmail A. GMC and the future of revalidation. Failure to act on good intentions. *BMJ* 2005; **330**: 1144–7.

39 Department of Trade and Industry. *360 Degree Feedback. Best Practice Guidelines.* www.cognology.biz/360bestprgdlns.pdf [accessed August 2006].

40 Farmer E A, Beard J, Dauphinee D, LaDuca T and Mann K. Assessing the performance of doctors in teams and systems. *Medical Education* 2002; **36**: 942–8.

41 Baker R. Commentary: can poorly performing doctors blame their assessment tools? *BMJ* 2005; **330**: 1254.

42 Evans R, Elwyn G and Edwards A. Review of instruments for peer assessment of physicians. *BMJ* 2004; **328**: 1240, doi:10.1136/bmj.328.7450.1240.

43 Hall W, Violato C, Lewkonia R, *et al.* Assessment of physician performance in Alberta: the physician achievement review. *Canadian Medical Association Journal* 1999; **161**: 52–6.

44 Elwyn G, Edwards A, Mowle S, *et al.* Measuring the involvement of patients in shared decision making: a systematic review of instruments. *Patient Education and Counseling* 2001; **43**: 5–22.

45 Wensing M, Elwyn G, Edwards A, Vingerhoets E and Grol R. Deconstructing patient centred communication and uncovering shared decision making: an observational study. *Medical Informatics and Decision Making* 2002; **2**: 2. Published on open-access publishing site, www.biomedcentral.com.

46 Mead N and Bower P. Patient-centredness: a conceptual framework and review of the empirical literature. *Social Science and Medicine* 2000; **51**: 1087–110.

47 Reznic R K, Regehr G, Yee G, Rothman A, Blackmore D and Dauphinee D. Process-rating forms versus task-specific checklists in an OSCE for medical licensure. *Academic Medicine* 1998; **73**: S97–9.

48 Schwatz M H, Colliver J A, Bardes C L, Charon R, Fried E D and Moroff S. Global ratings of videotaped performance versus global ratings of actions recorded in checklists: a criterion for performance assessment with standardized patients. *Academic Medicine* 1999; **74**: 1028–32.

49 Tate P, Foulkes J, Neighbour R, Campion P and Field S. Assessing physicians' interpersonal skills via videotaped encounters: a new approach for the Royal College of General Practitioners. *Journal of Health Communication* 1999; **4**: 143–52.

50 Pendleton D, Schofield T, Tate P and Havelock P. *The Consultation: An Approach to Learning and Teaching.* Oxford: Oxford University Press, 1984.

51 www.rcgp.org.uk/pdf/Exams_WBOOK06.pdf [accessed August 2006].

52 Campion P, Foulkes J, Neighbour R and Tate P. Patient centredness in the MRCGP video examination: analysis of large cohort. *BMJ* 2002; **325**: 691–2.

53 Look for examinations information on: www.rcgp.org.uk.

54 Cox J and Mulholland H. An instrument for assessment of videotapes of general practitioners' performance. *BMJ* 1993; **306**: 1043–6.

55 Fraser R C, McKinley R K and Mulholland H. Consultation competence in general practice: establishing the face validity of prioritised criteria in the Leicester assessment package. *BJGP* 1994; **44**: 109–13.

56 Fraser R C, McKinley R K and Mulholland H. Consultation competence in general practice: testing the reliability of the Leicester assessment package. *BJGP* 1994; **44**: 293–6.

57 McKinley R K, Dean P and Farooqi F. Reactions of volunteer general practitioners to educational assessment of their consultation performance: a qualitative study. *Education for Primary Care* 2003; **14**: 293–301.

58 Elwyn G, Edwards A, Wensing M, Hood K, Atwell C and Grol R. Shared decision making: developing the OPTION scale for measuring patient involvement. *Quality and Safety in Health Care* 2003; **12**: 93–9.

59 Elwyn G. OPTION scale manual. In: Shared decision making. Patient involvement in clinical practice. PhD thesis. University of Nijmegen, 2001, pp. 213–20.

60 Howie J G R, Heaney D J, Maxwell M and Walker J J. A comparison of a patient enablement instrument (PEI) against two established satisfaction scales as an outcome measure of primary care consultations. *Family Practice* 1998; **15**: 165–71.

61 Howie J G R, Heaney D J, Maxwell M, Walker J J, Freeman G K and Rai H. Quality at general practice consultations: cross sectional survey. *BMJ* 1999; **319**: 738–43.

62 Ogden J and Jain A. Patients' experiences and expectations of general practice: a questionnaire study of differences by ethnic group. *BJGP* 2005; **55**: 351–6.

63 CMO Report. *Good Doctors, Safer Patients.* London: DoH, 2006.

64 General Medical Council. *Good Medical Practice.* London: GMC, 1998.

The patient voice in doctors' learning

This chapter explores:

- the patient as expert and teacher – the need for new conversations
- the changing role of patients in doctors' learning ● learning with patients – practice development ● learning with patients – education and training
- the patient voice in the role of simulated patient (SP) ● learning from the patient voice – examples ● how to elicit and hear authentic patient voices
- GPs working with patients in education ● implications for the GP's role and sense of identity ● value of involving patients in doctors' learning.

'I started teaching as a patient because I wanted to make a difference to professionals. It's not always been easy. … I've learned so much myself. I feel valued and more confident as a person. I can negotiate with my own doctors better because I understand more about them and how they can change.'

ANDREA ARMITAGE
patient advocate, Senior Teaching Fellow in Communication Skills, Patient Perspective

'One of the most interesting discoveries of our work as Patients as Teachers was how to become a better patient. How could we have improved the experience?'

JOOLS SYMONS
carer advocate, Patients as Teachers facilitator and lead

'Patients no longer value bland reassurances, especially false ones. We want truth. And doctors who have learned to listen are beyond price.'

MITZI BLENNERHASSETT
patient advocate

We have discussed how roles and relationships are changing for professionals and patients. We have approached issues around the balance of power, control, authority and responsibility. How can patients and doctors learn to work together more effectively? In this chapter, we look at recent initiatives that involve patients in doctors' learning and explore what the patient voice offers to consultations in the 21st century.

By 'patient voice' we mean the active contribution into the learning of health professionals and service development by patients, carers and the community. This may be as: a patient or carer; expert patient; member of patient, carer or community group (or patient participation or patient/public involvement group); or as a properly prepared simulated patient. The term 'patient' is used here as shorthand also for other terms used in different settings: client; consumer; service user; survivor; the public.

The patient as expert and teacher: the need for new conversations

In their seminal study of GP consultations in London in the 1970s,[1] sociologist David Tuckett and his colleagues described the notion of patients as experts on their personal experience of illness and pointed out how their expertise is a necessary complement to doctors' expertise about disease when dealing with problems. They recommended that GPs should explore patients' experiential knowledge during the consultation. This is a prerequisite for the shared understanding and decision making we have discussed through this book. The notion can be hard for professionals to acknowledge, however, models viewing the patient as passive and lacking in knowledge, and the wider world of the patient as essentially irrelevant, still dominate early medical education.

Working *with* patients involves sharing power and responsibility. Despite training in consultation skills and a prevailing rhetoric of patient-centred care, many new British GPs have been unable to demonstrate significant levels of working with patients during recorded consultations for their College Membership (MRCGP) examination.[2] A recent study of primary care practitioners' management of menstrual disorders[3] suggests that GPs' capacity to work with patients can be limited by their need to 'achieve medical identity', which does not yet, for many doctors in their daily practice, include adopting shared decision making. Besides knowledge acquired through their experience, more patients now also have access, in our more highly educated society with its sophisticated consumerism, to wider medical and complementary medical ideas, via the internet and patients' groups. Some GPs, especially those younger or less sure of themselves, can find this threatening and overwhelming, rather than helpful.

Meanwhile, commentators[4] emphasise ever more strongly that the task of the health professional in the 21st century will be to help patients manage their own health and negotiate their professional role in that task. We recognise that involving patients in talking about, understanding and solving problems is not easy for many students and doctors – nor is it easy for patients. It entails a shift in perception and attitude, as well as behaviour. We would argue that it involves seeing patients as people with resources as well as deficits, capacities as well as pathology. This means regarding patients as capable of contributing to the exploration of problems – as worthy of partnership. It also means not making assumptions about patients' ideas and hopes, but rather putting energy into discovering these. It does not mean denying how vulnerable and needy patients can be, but rather finding a way to share the burden.

We have acknowledged some barriers for doctors in listening to patients, in particular anxieties about being overwhelmed, lack of time and loss of professional role. Is there a role for patients in helping professionals to overcome these? What needs to change in the way that patients behave with professionals? And what transformations can occur if patients and doctors work together differently?

To help doctors listen well to the patient voice, a key method has already been developed during the latter half of the 20th century: a great many people from our local communities contribute to professional education as SPs. Unfortunately, this proxy voice of the patient (also described in Chapter 7 and mentioned in other chapters of this book) has often been solely doctor directed, rather than patient centred. In the 21st century, there are widespread moves to bring the patient voice into co-teaching and assessment. The SP method, widely used in medical education, is an important focus for this. We will discuss further the need for authenticity in the portrayal of the patient and the need for processes to ensure the ethical and effective use of this method.

To learn how to relate differently, we need new conversations where different perspectives can be shared. This book describes the development of theory and practice in talking with patients and working together to solve problems. Already these ideas are being extended to encompass the changing roles of doctors and other professionals, and working on a daily basis in mixed teams, involving the patient. The notion of asking patients about their ideas and concerns during consultations has been a key force for bringing in the patient perspective. To cope with the current complexities and changes in health care, ideas have been offered for new ways of talking about problems, recognising the authority of different perspectives of team members, patients, families and carers.[5] Now, 'co-production' of health by patients, professionals and communities is being attempted in order to change not only health behaviours, but also the design of services, for example in diabetes care.[6] Surgeons in Austria have also used the notion of co-production when describing how patients can be supported to help ensure recuperation after surgery.[7]

Julian Tudor Hart, the GP who carried out important research with his local Welsh community, describes how:

> As a group, caring professionals have a long way to go before their relationships with patients always reach the quality they would like to receive when they themselves need care. Viewed not as consumers but as fellow workers in production of health, patients also have much to learn. When these two groups bring their skills together, both learn from each other to become more tolerant, thoughtful, effective, better informed and therefore more open to doubt. ... The real problem has been to achieve care systems that promote rather than impede sustained growth of these relationships, which develop naturally in consultations between equals.[8]

There are real difficulties for professionals while engaging with patients, arising partly from the pressures of modern health care and life. 'Difficult' patients seem more in evidence. We have found that some professionals now articulate more openly their fear of 'aggressive', 'angry', 'manipulative' or 'stupid' patients, given the shifting balances of power between them. We shall look more closely at how learning with a patient voice can address these issues to achieve a healthier outcome for all.

In this chapter, we will outline examples, highlighting the challenges thrown up by these fresh dialogues and the opportunities created for learning between professionals, between patients, and between patients and professionals.

The changing role of patients in doctors' learning

Patients' role in medical education has developed away from that of passive object of medical scrutiny, as a living or dead body. The patient's voice was silenced during the developments of early medical technologies. We described in Chapter 2 how the patient's account of illness again became recognised by leaders of the profession as core to diagnosis, even while technical processes were increasingly relied on to tell doctors what was going on. Some clinicians continue to be more comfortable with technicalities than with people, however, and this is the model they put across as teachers. We are all aware of the image of the patient lying in bed, ignored, while he or she is discussed by a consultant with students. Changes in our expectations of professional behaviour mean that more care is now taken to respect patients' vulnerabilities during such teaching ward rounds. But do clinical teachers also think patients have something to say from their own perspective that will really be helpful for medical learning?

Students can learn the value of listening to patients just by being with patients, of course, and all the more so since their education has included more patient contact in primary care. Here patients are up, dressed and in their own world, rather than prostrate in the world of the hospital. Recognising patients' potential for a more active contribution to student learning is a recent phenomenon: Wykurz and Kelly, educationalists in London medical schools, reviewed publications from the previous 30 years to identify the changing role of patients as teachers.[9] They found that learning from patients who had been prepared for teaching in their own right (not simply as audio-visual aids for clinicians) helped students to increase confidence, reduce anxiety and generate new insights. Others have built on this work: nursing students who engaged with active patient teachers were found to be more patient centred, less judgemental and less likely to stereotype patients.[10]

Our experience as educators of working with patients and the community confirms these effects, not only in student learning, but also in professional development. Earlier, Wykurz had argued that if patients are regarded as equal citizens in educating professionals, this shift in status will reflect the shift in attitudes of those leading the teaching.[11] For practitioners, working with patients in a fuller way can develop new understandings and relationships for service delivery; this is then modelled for their trainees and students. Further, we have found that the patient voice can challenge learners' assumptions and help them change their behaviour. We shall now unravel how this happens.

Learning with patients: practice development

In the UK, key government policy directives to involve patients and the public in the development of NHS services have increased the opportunities for professionals to learn from patients. While some efforts have been 'tick box' exercises, there has been some successful learning by organisations and there are lessons for those working in medical education with students and trainees.

Fisher and Gilbert involved local patients in helping a group of GP practices in London to develop their clinical guidelines for cardiac care and mental health.[12] The project leaders were experienced in developing community-based meetings, and set these up in such a way that patients and professionals were able to listen to each other. The professionals learnt a good deal more from their patients' feedback than just how to organise their services. They received positive feedback and suggestions, and learnt to take more account of patients' contribution to care. Their behaviour changed and local healthcare delivery improved.

Another programme, 'Preparing Professionals for Participation with the Public', also based in London, offers further insight into what is needed for successful learning from patients. It has been more fully described elsewhere:

> This programme aimed to help primary care professionals undertake change and shape a less hierarchical, more patient-focused organisation. It helped them examine their attitudes to patient involvement, critically appraise the culture within their practice team and open up to learning from patients.

Those who developed the programme identified the following stages to its success:

> First, it is important to give professionals the opportunity to explore anxieties about involving patients. The group often feels threatened and worried about being overwhelmed by patients' demands. The practice team can see itself joined against a common enemy that might be patients, the system or a government-imposed agenda. These feelings need to be expressed and understood.

> Second, it is useful to emphasise building upon what practices do already. This can be facilitated by:

> - encouraging positive reflection on the details of daily practice for the team

> - talking about enlarging the area of overlap between patients' needs and those of the practice

> - sharing good ideas.[13]

So successful learning with patients by practice teams involves safe opportunities to explore anxieties and to work from what they already do well. These professionals are then more likely to model and encourage openness to the patient's perspective for their trainees and students.

Learning with patients: education and training

This is an evolving field with good practice beginning to be shared and developed. The first international conference 'Where's the Patient Voice in Health Professional Education?' was held in Vancouver in 2005.[14] Patients, carers and community members met with health professional educators, researchers and students from many disciplines including medicine, nursing, pharmacy, occupational therapy and physiotherapy, social work, psychology and law. Ideas and successful strategies for tackling the barriers and challenges to involving patients effectively in professional education were shared. This was done through a process of 'appreciative inquiry', a powerful approach to addressing problems that focuses on what works and builds on successes, thus echoing the successful methods used in primary care development.

The conversations at this conference were also marked by their focus on equal collaboration: the conference summary report emphasises that 'Conference participants ignored traditional boundaries – the silos that keep them isolated – and focused on learning from each other no matter what their background or credentials.'[14]

Successful learning with patients in Australia, Canada, UK, USA and New Zealand included the following:

1 Patients contribute their experiential knowledge in teaching students how to perform a more accurate and gentle physical examination, and help them understand the impact of illness and disability on people's lives – also to share the hard-won strategies patients have discovered that help them cope with their challenges

2 Local people serve as simulated or standardised patients, helping students learn communication and other clinical skills, within a philosophy of collaboration

3 Patients participate as equal partners in research projects, not just as subjects, but also in determining the research questions

4 Patients sit on advisory groups or core committees, helping to define curricula of professional schools and training

5 Patients work in partnership with providers of community services, to make them more accessible and appropriate

6 Patients help improve health outcomes by developing self-help groups and sharing patients' expertise.

A number of issues about involving patients emerged. Patients and their organisations are eager to contribute and, when they do, learners say they learn more effectively. Many patients have identified personal benefits of involvement. Patients should be supported and rewarded appropriately for their contribution. The use of language in health care can have powerful effects and educators need to remain mindful of this, including the language used to describe patient involvement. This means saying 'working with' patients, rather than 'using' patients, for example. Interprofessional working and learning with a patient voice offer a way to understand all perspectives and their impact. A follow-up conference has been held in the UK and a network and website of resources established.[15]

The patient voice and the role of the SP

Learning skills with SPs is now ubiquitous in clinical education. It was recognised at the Vancouver conference that learning to hear the patient voice occurs in SP work when carried out within the philosophy of collaboration, which is what this chapter is chiefly concerned with. Given the growing part that SPs will be playing in teaching and assessment in health care, and the need for quality assurance and valid methods, it is becoming ever more vital to understand what constitutes ethical and effective SP work.

Simulated consultations are not game playing – in fact, the method is taken so seriously that it is used not only by the Royal College of General Practitioners, but also by the Royal Colleges of Physicians and of Surgeons, and by other medical licensing authorities all over the world. Work on developing this method with many leading practitioners in Manchester, Cambridge, Merseyside, London, Chicago and Leeds, as described earlier in this book, has shown how powerful a learning experience it can provide. There are many important questions about how that power is used, in what way patients are represented in simulations, and how learners and professionals are treated. Significant health resources in terms of human effort and money go into SP work. The crucial question is 'What makes a good SP experience?'

Background to the development of simulated patients
Some background is useful here (see also Chapter 7 for more information and note further comments on different forms of SP work in other chapters); a proxy patient voice has been provided in medical education in various ways. Before the introduction of SPs, role playing of patients by fellow students for their peers to practise communication with was common. It

remains a useful way for students, when 'being' the patient, to understand the patient perspective and experience. When students are successfully encouraged to portray a patient faithfully, or, indeed, be themselves for a role play interview as a patient, this can work well for the other learners too. But role playing with peers can be uncomfortable and students are often resistant. In the past, students would role play as the doctor as well, projecting themselves forward. However, it was found that students learnt best by being themselves and basing their role play in the context in which they are currently training.

An SP offers an opportunity for safe practice with someone from outside the peer group. Much like simulated flights for airline pilots, it is a rehearsal for real life, in a situation as near to real life as possible, where mistakes can be made and no one gets hurt. Attending to safety for all participants in SP exercises is vital to allow for experimentation. We explore later how to ensure this, so that the voice of the patient and of the person in SPs and learners is respected and mutual understanding achieved.

When SPs were first established in the UK in the late 1970s the work was undertaken by community theatre members who were closely linked to local patients, and had their own practice in group work and learning with the local community. Developed collaboratively with leading GP teachers, this SP practice emphasises the role of the lay voice in creating patient roles and giving feedback.[16] Earlier work in the USA and Canada described working with doctors' notes of patients to train local people, sometimes actors, to simulate as closely as possible a patient case.[17] In the UK, we came to understand that this would incorporate only a medical view, missing out on a patient perspective, which is vital not only for content but also for effective portrayal of the patient and feedback. So, patient roles would first be outlined by doctors from their experience of a patient case, but would later be adapted with the SP.

Later work in the USA was with 'patient instructors', patients with chronic illness who portrayed their own case and who were trained to assess the consultation skills of medical students. This work did have a patient voice, as we observed while visiting this scheme, but the contribution of this voice was not credited – rather, the stress was placed on the fact that local doctors had monitored the case outlines and agreed the criteria for assessment. This sanctioning by the doctors did allow for the lone assessment, one to one, of students by the patients, which gave them a powerful role and was copied during a successful experiment to promote working with patients in UK medical education.[18]

The various styles of SP work were brought together in the USA during the establishment of medical accreditation and assessment methods requiring standardisation, so SP in the USA now more often stands for 'standardised patient' and standardised patient is the term increasingly used elsewhere for assessments, such as objective structured clinical examinations (OSCEs) and simulated surgeries (see also Chapter 8). However, recent discussions with other practitioners have shown that many of us feel that it is more difficult to achieve an effective patient voice in much of this standardised work [19,20] and so its validity is being questioned. Certainly, notions of standardisation of SP roles for experiential learning can be misguided, as they do not allow for the necessary flexibility of response by the SP.

The development of SP work is uneven; sometimes it is still done by enlisting non-clinical staff from the institution involved on an *ad hoc* basis to role play patients, or actors from agencies with equally little preparation or training. This work is usually ineffective and can be reliably used only to train set skills by rote. It is hardly applicable for learning how to navigate the complex relationships in health care and does not have validity or reliability for assessment.

Evaluating SP work

As demonstrated in the learning examples below, good SP work is not about teaching superficial 'people management' techniques that are primarily for the benefit of GPs and their staff; these can best be taught through much simpler, more economical formats. Rather, this work is for the benefit of *patients* and for the long-term development of better consultations as a whole, which ultimately will also be more productive and satisfying for GPs.

In evaluating this work the key questions are: 'What will increase the confidence of the learner (GP, registrar, student) to listen, and not to feel diminished?' 'What will give the learner an authentic experience of the diverse voices of our communities?' 'What will make sure that such learning addresses the necessary and complex task of developing a collaborative approach with patients, with which this book is concerned?' 'How can SPs contribute a valid voice to the training and assessment of health professionals, rather than act merely as an audio-visual aid to reflect professionals' perceptions?' 'Who should ensure the integrity of this?'

One way of answering these questions is to highlight the issue of respect. This is the essential element in a collaborative relationship. However, this issue raises still more questions. How do you teach respect? How do we learn to respect patients in a world that often teaches the opposite? How can we structure training and accreditation to nurture respect? It is crucial for successful learning and collaboration with patients that doctors respect patients, patients respect doctors, and teachers/facilitators respect learners and patients. There are moves to establish accreditation procedures for

SPs:[21] an effective patient voice in this will be vital to ensure such respect and thus 'fit-for-purpose' accreditation of medical practice, in which SPs will be heavily involved.

Essential steps to effective SP work: recruitment and preparation, structures for learning, patient role development, safety issues, feedback and support

Processes to ensure valid patient voices and effective SP work are still developing and some of our understandings have still not been articulated. The study of SP practice, particularly in relation to theories of learning and of performance, is ongoing. Some of the necessary steps have been identified, however. First, much attention needs to be given to recruitment and selection. People should be recruited from a wide base, and carefully. This means making every effort to include people with the appropriate patient experience, both to be SPs and to help in the training of SPs and the development of SP roles. So an SP role of a drug addict, for example, would be based on the experience of those who do admit to drug addiction problems and/or those close to them, and not only on doctors' views of this.

SPs need to be people with some self-understanding. What is the benefit for the potential SP? It is important that he or she is not motivated by a personal interest in achieving shock effects, receiving vicarious attention, manipulating others, or retaliating against doctors. Most SPs become involved because they want to develop personally and to make a contribution, to do something worthwhile. If they are actors, the best people are those who put representing patients well first, and only secondarily are interested in relating this to their professional practice. Some actors have to unlearn being mouthpieces for set scripts. They may find it as hard to empathise with the seldom-heard voices from our communities as do some health professionals who outline patient roles. Many sorts of people can make good SPs: it is also often better to employ people with long-term conditions, or carers, or members of community groups so that the mutual learning and employment opportunities feed back more directly into the local area.

Next, in effective SP preparation, they are encouraged to spend time listening to each other and to patients; this might be in groups discussing patients' learning journeys, for example (as described in this chapter). It can help when people come from patient and carer self-help groups where people meet to talk to each other already. Again, awareness is a key issue for potential SPs: they need to learn to be aware of others' experience, but also to acknowledge what it is that resonates with their own experience. In preparing to play a drug addict, for example, a trainee SP, even if lacking familiarity with the world of drug addiction or alcoholism, would be encouraged to identify in what areas of their own life they are touched by an experience of addiction, of whatever sort. It is that identification which enables the SP to work from a place of understanding, of both themselves and of the patient they play, rather than from a place of denial that can lead to the projection, at arm's length, of stereotypes and caricatures. It is a mantra of medical education that learners should put themselves into patients' shoes; the intention is that SPs should do just that, in order to help learners.

What constitutes good facilitation with an SP: structures for feedback

Learners usually practise talking with SPs in small groups, with feedback, which should include feedback from the person role playing the patient. To make the most of the SP resource, learners should have the opportunity to experiment with different approaches, both in response to their own reflection on how an interaction went and also to feed back from the SP and peers and facilitators in the room. Freire, the influential Brazilian educator and community developer, argued that real learning only occurs through a process of dialogue between teachers and other learners, based on mutual respect.[22] In this way, learners and teachers are involved in an active and equal relationship in which both parties learn from each other. We see a parallel with this process and that of the new conversations mooted during this chapter. In both processes, ways forward are constantly negotiated; there is no one right answer and the final responsibility and decision rest with the learner/patient.

This understanding of the learner during the SP method means that learners need to be encouraged to venture into new territory. It is risky, interviewing in public, often about sensitive matters. Where the role-played encounter will go is unknown to all present. We find the writings of the child psychologist Bowlby useful for understanding why clear structures must be in place for 'a safe space from which exploration is possible'.[23] Learners must be enabled to identify their real strengths, then use and build on these to respond to difficulties discovered by themselves or others. SPs who bring a patient voice understand how this works; theirs is the most powerful voice in the room.

The role of the facilitator in these sessions is to hold learners in a safe structure for debriefing and feedback.

Too often, though, comments made by others during such sessions are given in a rote, perfunctory fashion that does not encourage real dialogues and honest reflection. Participants, sometimes because they do not feel safe, may be hidebound by ideas of what they are supposed to say and do, rather than applying the careful 'work of attention' to what is actually happening in front of them.[24]

> **Box 9.1 ○ A structure for debriefing and feedback for interviews with SPs**
>
> (This section was developed with Jerry Henry and Mike Forrest of Merseyside Postgraduate GP Education.)
>
> ① The learner reflects on the interaction and what they may need help with.
>
> ② The learner identifies what went well, checking assumptions with the SP, who remains in role.
>
> ③ The group helps the learner to identify strengths, again checking with the SP.
>
> ④ The learner further identifies areas to revisit, generates alternative approaches and rehearses and evaluates these with the SP.
>
> ⑤ The group helps with the above process.
>
> ⑥ The SP comes out of role and makes any further comments.
>
> ⑦ The learner summarises his or her learning.

Of course, this is also the core challenge for the learner too when talking with the patient. The patient, as in Freire's model of learning and development, has to be part of defining the problem in order to take an active role in finding a solution. Professionals at all stages of learning need confidence to apply their own clinical expertise whilst facilitating the patient's involvement. Confidence building entails engaging with the person in the professional, showing respect to their perspective and offering, transparently, others' perspectives.

Professional educators also have to learn how to be open to the still unknown in order to model this demanding task for learners. In the SP method, this would mean not writing a 'script' for the SP. (This risks stereotyping patients, leaving out the perspective of the person playing the role. This person, in turn, must be open and able to give voice to the person within a patient role.) Rather, a role must be created or refined in collaboration with the SP. It would also mean, wherever possible, that the patient voice is engaged in the development of SP roles and the whole learning process.

Safety and aggressive, violent patients

The SP method is not appropriate for addressing the extreme situations involving aggressive and violent people that can arise for professionals raised in Chapter 5. As in the real-life situation, certain clear boundaries need to be established. In real life these would be panic buttons, awareness of escape routes, body language and so on. This can be discussed in much more straightforward and less costly ways than working with SPs. As shown in examples later, professionals' fears about this can affect their attitude to the majority of patients who may be merely upset or (sometimes justifiably) cross. So at the beginning of SP work to do with addressing difficulties with anger, it is helpful to clarify briefly at the start what can be put in place to deal with extreme cases. This helps learners deal with what is in front of them, rather than with their fearful fantasy.

The development of patient roles for learning

There are various approaches to developing patient roles with SPs, some more successful than others. SPs should be encouraged to start out with role-playing situations that are close to their own experience; in this person-centred approach the SP is taken as a starting point and, ideally, stories are built around them. This is distinct from an amateur-dramatics approach, which is dependent on costume and props, and acting a 'character'. Rather, it is a process of the SP reaching a point of veracity within themselves from which they find the voice of the patient they are role playing; they can then respond intuitively 'in the moment' during the simulation with the learner and thus give authentic feedback. In this way, when talking as the patient to the doctor/student, they carry the conviction needed to enable the learner to gain insight, to change behaviour and to question deep-set attitudes and beliefs. Many doctors have found that such an experience with an SP was a turning point for them.[25]

This approach is at its most powerful when designed with learners at the time of the SP session. Students can identify what they feel they need to address and the SP, working from the patient perspective, then creates a role that will address that learning need and will resonate with their own authentic experience.

SPs can also successfully adapt 'off the peg' patient role outlines or briefs for learners and bring in their own acknowledged experience to adapt the role where necessary, interpreting its meaning and providing authenticity.

Preparing a role – example

In this example, the SP worked from the learners' brief, provided by a GP for doctors in practice. Box 9.2.

The SP here had to carefully feel her way into an authentic portrayal of a patient who has displayed manipulative, even criminal, behaviour. In order to give effective feedback she has to be able to empathise with the person she is role playing. She thought about people she knew and about her own experience: What might drive this patient to become addicted to diazepam? How could that feeling of addiction lead on to stealing and more risk taking? What would help her to stop? The GP had originally based this role on a

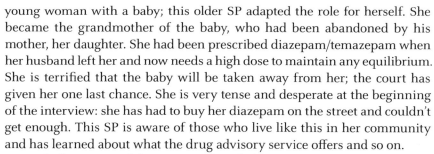

Box 9.2 ○ Sharon Edwards – a brief for learners

Sharon was seen as a temporary resident one week ago, requesting prescription for diazepam. Advised to register with practice; no prescription can be given till previous patient notes arrive.

Notes have now arrived: she is 53 years' old, unemployed, living in temporary council accommodation. She has a five-year history of diazepam/temazepam use. Seen by drugs advisory service in other area, but defaulted on a number of appointments; discharged after selling drugs on the street. Surgery staff suspected she may have altered the quantity on some of her prescriptions.

Last entry 6 weeks ago: 'Due in court tomorrow on charge of credit card fraud, thinks she may get custodial sentence. Tearful, requests diazepam to help get her through.'

You, as a GP in this practice, will now be meeting Sharon for the first time (she saw a colleague of yours last time).

young woman with a baby; this older SP adapted the role for herself. She became the grandmother of the baby, who had been abandoned by his mother, her daughter. She had been prescribed diazepam/temazepam when her husband left her and now needs a high dose to maintain any equilibrium. She is terrified that the baby will be taken away from her; the court has given her one last chance. She is very tense and desperate at the beginning of the interview: she has had to buy her diazepam on the street and couldn't get enough. This SP is aware of those who live like this in her community and has learned about what the drug advisory service offers and so on.

We shall now unpick how SPs work with their careful preparation of roles to provide effective learning. This patient case had social difficulties and mental health problems: people who admit to these kind of difficulties can help SPs develop roles, as described below, but it is also possible for good SPs to draw on their own experience for this. For example, the SP playing Sharon thought about a close relative with stigmatising mental health problems and ensuing poor behaviour, and how people found it hard to see his good points and thus understand how to help him move on. This gave her insight into how Sharon could be helped to move on, once she feels enough safety and trust with the GP, and vice versa.

Giving feedback in and out of role

Good SPs have clear ideas about how best to give their feedback to learners:

> I stay in role during most of the feedback, speaking directly as the patient. This means I let the learner know my responses, rather than report on them, as it were. It means we can keep on talking together in the room. It makes it easier for the learner to re-try approaches.

Another SP offers more about giving feedback in and out of role:

It's multilayered. There's a lot of feedback to give in role, about what I felt and feel about how the interviewer behaves. Sometimes, depending on how the discussion is unfolding, I reveal, rather than baldly report, how something has affected me. The learner can try out a new approach and then we look together at how that went. Often, at the end, if the facilitator has worked with me well, when I come out of role there is nothing else to say about what has happened. I then step back and may offer a comment to the group about the whole discussion. Usually I say something supportive about the way they have been discussing things to help their group work. Sometimes, my personal experience as a carer can offer something extra, particularly when working with interprofessional groups. I can say: ask me anything you want – I'm supported in a well-facilitated group, they're supported and we can talk about things we just couldn't broach while in the clinic.

Good SPs know their practice in a way that someone who has not been an SP cannot. Their insights have been left out of too much SP activity. Or, their efforts are there, making the learning happen, but they are not recognised and therefore cannot be built on.

Learning from a patient voice: examples

We will now look at examples of learning from a patient voice in more detail. These are real examples of learning processes, taken from notes at the time and reflections afterwards.

Example: learning to work with patients – overcoming assumptions and stereotypes

A group of GPs attending a Fresh Start course[26] run for the London Postgraduate Deanery were working on communication issues for primary care teams with an SP and a facilitator. There had been discussion of their anxieties about dealing with 'difficult', 'demanding,' 'angry' patients. The SP who worked with them uses a patient perspective approach, developing his role from an empathic understanding of the person he will role play. He became the father of a 15-year-old girl who has been prescribed the contraceptive pill. He has arrived at the surgery, insisting on seeing a doctor, to protest. In the scenario, the prescribing GP is away from the surgery today. The receptionist has telephoned one of his colleagues to say that the father is at her desk with a complaint. A volunteer GP from the learning group agrees to act as the colleague and meet him.

The father asks the volunteer GP why his daughter was prescribed the pill, what did they think they were doing – 'She's 15, 15! Are you allowed to prescribe without me knowing?' The volunteer is careful not to compromise the daughter's confidentiality and does not confirm the prescription, but attempts to reason with the father: 'Would you rather she got pregnant?'

During the debrief after the role play, the volunteer reflected that his approach did not calm the father down. In fact, the father became more agitated. He was then invited to identify his strengths: protecting confidentiality of the daughter as patient, while negotiating with her father, also a patient. The SP, still in role, gave him feedback: 'I appreciated you agreeing to see me and felt you were really paying attention to me. I just can't bear to think of my daughter, on the pill or pregnant, at 15. …'

The group then talked of their own reactions should this situation happen in their own families: one GP, a father, said he understood how the father felt. Another, a mother, said that the father had to accept reality: 15 was a later age for sexual experience than for many of the families she worked with; his daughter needed protection from pregnancy and the legal situation was that the father could do nothing about it. Others in the group wondered about the daughter's mother – where was she in the picture?

They also shared how the father's first entrance had made them feel: anxious and fearful for the volunteer, because of the father's anger. They were invited to reflect on what evidence they had for his anger. They identified the unusual nature of his demand to see a doctor without an appointment, his assertiveness and the challenge to their practice, his exclamations about his daughter's age. The SP is a tall, well-built, white, working-class Londoner who seems typical of some of the patients that these GPs see. This group of GPs originate mainly from other cultures, reflecting the changing nature of the population of GPs in the UK's inner cities.

'He's angry. I'd want to be careful' said one. 'I think rather he is upset. I think I would be too' said another.

The volunteer GP then reconsidered his approach to the patient: perhaps he had worked himself up to defend the practice and could not listen to the father's distress.

He then returns to the role play with the SP and reflects back his understanding of the father's distress. Immediately, the father is less tense and more hesitant and thoughtful, as he focuses on the pain he is feeling about his daughter. He talks about how the girl's mother knew about the situation and his bewilderment on finding a packet of the daughter's pills. The SP fed back again after the role play: 'You've helped me think about it more clearly.'

Others from the group then took the simulated consultation further, continuing to explore with the father what was going on and how the situation could be improved. It was made clear what the practice's responsibilities were: paying attention to the boundaries of confidentiality; the law about under-age prescribing; and the need to help young women avoid unwanted pregnancy. They also gave attention to the father's distress, trying out the kind of questions that could help him to reflect and move on. The father acknowledged that he felt cut out of the picture by both daughter and mother, and was trying to get back in control. Perhaps he had to let go. … One offered to meet him again, with the mother and/or daughter.

The group then wondered how much they had made assumptions about this person. They previously had a stereotype of an angry patient in mind that had stopped them working with him effectively. In this way of learning, they were able to counteract the stereotype and could be open to addressing the issues for the father, and for his family. This was important to do, not only to defuse a complaint against the practice, but also for the good of the patients. There was a question of patient safety here, as well as practice safety: awareness was needed about keeping an eye on the father's need for control and so on.

This simulation, with someone able to portray a 'difficult' patient from within his perspective, gave these GPs a chance to grapple with an authentic patient problem and voice. This is not the same as learning techniques of manipulation to manage patients whom doctors find difficult. People who play doctor-devised roles of 'angry' patients, without a view and understanding from within those patients, may not offer a real learning opportunity. Everyone involved may be acting out assumptions, stereotypes and fantasies. The SP who has not developed their own role carefully, with respect and empathy for the person they are portraying, is unlikely to be authentically responsive to the actual interaction and less able to allow doctors to realise the true effects of their behaviour and attitude. This is a deeper level of learning than mere skills practice.

Patients learn from this work too and there are health benefits to their explicit involvement, as the Vancouver conference identified. That is why at Leeds University and elsewhere there have been efforts to widen participation from the local community in the group of SPs who contribute to students' learning and a growing commitment to prepare them well for using their own voice.[27] Empathy and respect are more likely to be found in patient teachers who come from similar backgrounds to the people they portray and who are supported to trust their own perceptions and speak up.

The next examples explore other ways that the patient voice contributes to professional learning. After these, we will look more closely at how this is done and consider its advantages.

Example: patients helping to shape and validate patient-focused interprofessional learning

Students of nursing, physiotherapy, occupational therapy, medicine, social work, midwifery and dietetics are brought together in sessions held in their clinical workplaces, towards the end of their education at Leeds University. They work with the Patients as Teachers group to explore the patient's journey and to examine the different professional roles taken with the patient and their carer(s).[28]

The patient voice is now introduced at an earlier stage of the learning process: patients are invited to shape and validate the learning materials for these sessions, including the creation of the SP roles. Outlines of potential SP roles are circulated to a wide, multiprofessional team of clinical facilitators for comment. A workshop is then held with some of the clinical teachers together with patients, most of whom have long-term conditions and have been prepared and supported to speak their mind with professionals in a constructive way (see below for more about this preparation).

The development of a role about a woman with diabetes illustrates the particular contribution the patient voice can make:

> The original draft for the role, by a clinician, describes a patient who has had diabetes for 14 years and who sometimes forgets to give herself insulin or gives herself the wrong amount. She has just become pregnant but is unaware of the complications for her baby or herself that this may bring. The students' tasks, when interacting with an SP in this role, would be to ensure that the patient 'is fully aware of her responsibilities during and after the pregnancy to ensure a healthy mother and baby'. They are also expected to establish her 'willingness and ability to comply' and awareness of the large multiprofessional team who will need to be involved in her care.

The patients in the group were uneasy about this SP role, as drafted. In small groups they explored with the clinicians an alternative view:

> Has she forgotten her insulin or mistaken the dosage (after 14 years' experience of diabetes?), or does she make a conscious decision not to comply? Some patients want to establish a balance in how they manage their condition and may take the informed decision to take the minimum medicine to avoid danger. Is it likely that she is entirely unaware of diabetic complications in pregnancy? Should not the emphasis be on finding out what she understands and what her perspective is? Should not the emphasis also be on what advice or resources the patient needs to help her cope with managing her illness, rather than telling her about her

responsibilities as conceived by the health professional team?

The role was redeveloped to be more concerned with shared decision making, recognising that, while the patient needs to be fully informed, she may not comply. In the first draft, the shared decision making was about the professionals sharing *their* decisions with each other.

The patient perspective had brought an appreciation of the patient's expertise, a process described in more depth earlier. Of course, there are patients who cannot remember dosages and so on. Such a patient role could be developed with patients who are themselves in the situation of forgetting. For example, such work has been developed at St George's Medical School in London, in another context, with the help of people with learning difficulties.[29] The point is that students in the 21st century need guidance to help them respect and work with patients' capacities. Patients' input into shaping and validating learning materials helps ensure that this is not forgotten.

At the end of this workshop, the patients and clinicians reflected together on its outcomes. The patients' input had been drawn from their own experience of long-term conditions – not only of diabetes – and they had shared this, for example their own lack of compliance and its consequences. They felt taking part in such a discussion is a demanding process: 'This takes a lot; you have to give from your whole self.'

Some of the clinicians then shared how they had held back some of their personal experiences, partly because they were painful and partly because they were not sure of the ground rules. Should they (the professionals) be talking of personal experiences? It was felt that it was important for these feelings to be acknowledged, i.e. for the patient voice within the professional to be recognised. Ground rules and frameworks for dealing with feelings throughout the process were needed – there is a parallel with looking after students' feelings. It was agreed that the patient voice within the professional was an important complement to, though not a substitute for, the independent patient voice and that the clinicians should share as much or as little of their personal experience as they felt comfortable with.

Example: learning with patients about end-of-life decision making

The staff at a hospice in Leeds wanted to make a training video for primary care colleagues about end-of-life decision making, and in particular 'do not resuscitate' orders (DNRs). They wanted to help professionals to have conversations with patients about their preferences about resuscitation in advance so that, for example, if a patient in a terminal stage were to suffer a cardiac arrest in an ambulance, the paramedics would have a clear instruction from the patient about their preferences. They asked the Leeds University School of Medicine's communication team to help with the training.

They were encouraged to begin by exploring patients' views. A member of the Patients as Teachers group, who came from a local Cancer Support Network, facilitated a group discussion for patients and carers. These were people who had been touched by the issue, either in the past or in anticipation: one carer of her husband with cancer came with him in mind, but then remembered how resuscitation had been attempted on her mother in her nursing home. There had been little hope of its success, but, in the absence of a DNR, staff had felt bound to try and the woman felt her mother had had an unnecessarily undignified death. The group explored the difficulty of talking about, even thinking about, what a DNR order means.

The record of this meeting informed the learning process: another Patients as Teachers member, who had trained to be an SP, developed the role of a patient with whom the hospice doctor needed to discuss DNRs and this formed part of the training video, together with both their reflections on their discussion. The Patients as Teachers facilitator returned to the patient and carer group. They discussed the impact on them of exploring their own assumptions and preferences around end-of-life decisions. It had exposed a knowledge gap: for some, their ideas about resuscitation had come mainly through hospital medical dramas. They realised they had a concept of 'magic paddles' that could bring people back to life, even if they had cancer. They appreciated the opportunity to learn from each other and to prepare to make informed choices about DNRs, and they were pleased to help professional training. The learning journey had encompassed a wider group than just the health professionals.

How to elicit and hear authentic patient voices

By having a chance to reflect on our own experiences we can voice our fears and concerns, and discover whether we are in the right place in our journey to engage in working in partnership with healthcare professionals. This can help avoid the misunderstanding that here is a chance to blame all healthcare professionals for our past experiences.

JOOLS SYMONS
carer advocate, Patients as Teachers facilitator and lead

How do you prepare patients to enable them to contribute effectively to professionals' learning? We have found that inviting patient and community groups to lecture medical students or GP registrars can provide access to personal stories and testimonies of experiences with health professionals. But sometimes this gives the students and registrars a dispiriting view of professionals' capacity to help, without a vision of a new kind of role for doctors, based on collaborating with others. There is also the risk of voyeurism, exploitation of patients' pain and the 'burnout' of people who tell their stories repeatedly. How should we frame the patient voice in our teaching?

At Leeds University, there is a developing programme of engagement with local community groups during which there is evaluation of different approaches to working with the patient voice. One approach is based on exploring the patient's 'learning journey' in a small-group induction lasting three sessions:

> During the first session we talk about why we are in the room, what brought us here, why we want to be involved. A lot of my experiences with health professionals have been very positive and I want to give something back. On the other hand, I experienced a number of painful and traumatic consultations, and these have had a lasting effect. These were mainly due to lack of, or poor, communication between professionals and my partner and/or me, or professionals with each other. I want to feed this back and help ensure it doesn't happen to others. Many people in these groups feel like this.

Participants then take it in turns to tell their stories:

> All learning journeys are unique but yet there seem to be common themes. This commonality helps to build the group and develop a supportive atmosphere. Through this process we are able to identify and document these common themes in what we have learned from our experiences – about ourselves, about others, about the system. Then, in the next session, we begin to refocus and think about how those experiences could have been improved and how we can help deliver that message.

In the final session, participants look at how they could contribute – in teaching and/or the development of materials and/or joining curriculum committees – and assess whether they are ready to turn their experience into positive learning for others.

> It is a rare opportunity when healthcare students/professionals get the chance to celebrate what they do well and I think building on the positives is the way forward – do we really learn by constant criticism?

Recently, educators have worked in partnership with the new patient movements, such as expert patients and mental health service user groups, to establish structures and methods for ethical and effective patient involvement in health professional education and training. User-led services in mental health have been developed and subsequently user-lecturers have been appointed in university healthcare departments. O'Neill from Leeds calls for universities to take a strategic approach so that health professional teachers can work with patients as teachers. She describes layers of involvement, from token, to limited, to full engagement and partnership.[30] The Mental Health in Higher Education group (mhhe) in the UK has analysed the framework and support needed to make sure users can contribute well.[31] These principles apply when GPs work with patients at their practices and learn with patients or SPs for their own development as GPs, or during undergraduate or registrar education.

In Box 9.3 we outline principles for overcoming obstacles to professionals and students hearing the patient's voice (adapted from Morris and Trafford, who described work in primary care in London). The aim is to help professionals to learn to move towards a constructive dialogue with patients.

Box 9.3 ○ Ways of overcoming obstacles to hearing the patient's voice

① Preparing patients and professionals for partnership; give both parties a voice to express their creative ideas and difficult feelings.

② Involve patients near the beginning of any learning or development exercise, to help set the agenda.

③ Give opportunities to reflect on personal practice and experiment with new ways of seeing and behaving.

④ Establish clear structures to encourage a feeling of safety and openness to change.

⑤ Encourage professionals, students and patients to support each other to build on their strengths. This parallels and reinforces an empowerment model for individual patients.

⑥ Make sure that agreed outcomes from shared learning and development are jointly evaluated and followed up.

GPs working with patients in education

Recent developments in this field of work were reflected when a group of GP educators met at the Royal College of General Practitioners for an 'away-day' about focusing on developing a 'patient-led NHS'.[32] They discussed how new ways of working, making links and learning with others are becoming necessary in primary care. They felt patients could be allies in creating fresh educational approaches for new services. They outlined some immediate opportunities for learning with and from patients, not only for themselves as GPs, but also for their trainees, registrars and students.

Positive steps they recommended included:

- involve the voluntary sector in the design of service delivery – in the UK, this would be practice-based commissioning

- invite expert patients, patients who help other patients learn about self-care, as teachers and resources for vocational training groups

- ensure patient feedback is included in workplace assessments for practitioners, trainees, registrars and students

- involve patients in practice-based discussions with the team, trainees, registrars and students about their 'patient journey', taking into account their own efforts and community resources

- include feedback for learners from the patients in the assessment of assignments and case studies about patient-centred care.

Implications for the GP's role and sense of identity

I have to admit – if a patient goes against my clinical opinion, I feel rejected. So you think you know better than me? Why did you come to see me? You're wasting my time.

FRESH START COURSE PARTICIPANT

The World Health Organization argues for a recasting of roles and relationships in primary health care – this is in the context of the care of long-term conditions, with pressure on professionals to encourage self-management by patients and to ensure their information needs are met.[33] Already a number of steps have been taken along this road:

Important changes in policy and practice are slowly transforming the way that services are provided. All health professionals are challenged to expand their skills to meet the new complexities and challenges, particularly in the care of long-term conditions. A focus on the personal needs and expectations of individuals and how they manage their disease and live their lives, often with minimal intervention from health professionals, has helped to challenge dominant views that patients are passive and in some way lacking in knowledge and expertise. Traditional educational approaches are limited in their support of those who must shape the new world of primary care. Patient voices bring diversity into the teaching team and model the principle that patients and professionals need to appreciate each other's different but equally valuable expertise in order to build relationships and learn together.[34]

However, this is not simply a matter of consultation and communication skills education and training, but of cultural change. When responsibilities are shared, roles change. Therefore, behaviour and attitudes need to change and this can be difficult.[35] However, those GPs who have learned to do this find it very satisfying.[36] Today's GPs have been trained, by and large, for a different world from the one they now work in. The GP educators described earlier hoped that working with patients would help sustain the professional values they felt are under threat, i.e. those of personal care and autonomous professional judgement. But the implications of the patient voice raise another idea of the GP role and sense of identity, based on mutual learning and shared decision making. It is argued by some that modern medicine no longer involves professionals merely holding knowledge, but interpreting, engaging with and sharing knowledge – and uncertainty. This is not something that people can learn to do alone[37] but will need to do with support from others, in new conversations with fresh voices.

The expert patient ○ *reflections*

I can well remember the arrogance of youth: my first years as a doctor. While I was humble and self-effacing before my superiors (other doctors), in my persona as 'doctor' with patients I certainly did not always ask their opinions. At a basic level the patient's voice is expressed when doctors ask the patient his or her ideas about the illness (i.e. the patient-centred approach). Sometimes patients or relatives volunteer these ideas spontaneously. I remember the husband of one elderly lady, when I was a GP trainee, suggesting that his wife had lockjaw. She had cut her toe in the garden the day before and was now having difficulty speaking. He was right and she was treated for tetanus (and survived). But the concept of the expert patient involves more than listening to patients' ideas on their own health. Educators and clinicians need to involve patients actively in education and curriculum development, and seek their opinions on health service delivery. Once we nurture an environment in which patients' views are important, then as doctors we will learn so much about our own practice and improve our performance.

Box 9.4 ○ **Value of involving patients in doctors' learning**

This builds on the work by Wykurz and Kelly.

For doctors/learners

1. Access to personal experience and knowledge of health and illness.
2. Access to personal experience and knowledge of use of services.
3. Access to skills and strategies that patients develop to manage their own health.
4. Opportunity to rehearse skills and strategies.
5. Opportunity for constructive feedback.
6. Reduces anxiety.
7. Deepens understanding.
8. Increases confidence.
9. Improves skills and performance.
10. Increases respect for patients.
11. Influences attitudes and behaviour.
12. Places learning in context.
13. Uses authentic learning models, not based on stereotypes of patients, models partnership.
14. Opportunity to interact with seldom-heard voices.

For patients

15. Uses their knowledge about health, illness and their condition positively.
16. Increases their knowledge.
17. Acknowledges their expertise.
18. Creates a sense of empowerment.
19. Provides an opportunity to help future patients and professionals.
20. Provides new insights.
21. Improves their understanding of doctors.
22. Increases their faith in medical training and thus in professionals.
23. Enables them to take more part in consultations with professionals.
24. Provides opportunities for personal and professional development.
25. Provides employment for people with long-term conditions and others.

For learning organisations

26. Provides ways to improve services and support health professionals.
27. Provides access to patient voices to influence service development.
28. Enables educational institutions to fulfil their remit to link with local communities.

For patient and carer groups and other community organisations

29. Acknowledges community resources.
30. Provides ways to improve services and support patients.
31. Provides further resources for communities.

○ **Summary**

- Patients have something new to add in conversations about health care.

- Patients and the community can contribute to new understandings and delivery of health care.

- Learning with patients works for many professionals, in different ways.

- There are key principles to this working well.

- Preparing patients, real or simulated, is key, as is preparing professionals.

- GPs will need to consider afresh the way they view their role and responsibilities.

- Patients need to do this too – and they benefit.

○ **Acknowledgements**

The SPs whose work is quoted from in this chapter are:

- Ernie Dalton, co-founder of Spanner Workshops, SP trainer

- Rita Hunt, role player for Fresh Start Simulations, who works with Peter Burrows and Anwar Khan

- Jools Symons, lead for Patients as Teachers, SP, facilitator

- Sue Power, member of Spanner Workshops.

REFERENCES

1 Tuckett D, Boulton M, Olson C and Williams A. *Meetings between Experts. An Approach to Sharing Ideas in Medical Consultations.* London: Tavistock Publications, 1985.

2 Campion P, Foulkes J, Neighbour R and Tate P. Patient-centredness in the MRCGP examination: analysis of large cohort. *BMJ* 2002; **325**: 691–2.

3 Flynn N and Britten N. Does the achievement of medical identity limit the ability of primary care practitioners to be patient-centred? A qualitative study. *Patient Education and Counseling* 2006; **60**: 49–56.

4 Hasman A, Coulter A and Askham J. *Education for Partnership: Developments in Medical Education.* Oxford: Picker Institute, 2006.

5 Steinberg D. *Complexity in Healthcare and the Language of the Consultation*. Oxford: Radcliffe, 2005.

6 Cottam H and Leadbetter C. RED paper 01 *Health: Co-creating Services*. London: Design Council, 2004.

7 Trummer U, Mueller U, Nowak P, Stidl T and Pelikan J. Does physician–patient communication that aims at empowering patients improve clinical outcome? A case study. *Patient Education and Counseling* 2006; **61** (2): 299–306.

8 Tudor Hart J. *The Political Economy of Health Care: A Clinical Perspective*. Cambridge: Polity Press, 2006.

9 Wykurz G and Kelly D. Developing the role of patients as teachers: literature review. *BMJ* 2002; **325**: 818–21.

10 Forrest M, Risk G, Masters T and Brown G. Mental health service user involvement in nurse education: exploring the issues. *Journal of Psychiatric and Mental Health Nursing* 2000; **7**: 51–7.

11 Wykurz G. Patients in medical education: from passive participants to active partners. *Medical Education* 1999; **33**: 634–6.

12 Fisher B and Gilbert D. Patient involvement in clinical effectiveness. In: Gillam S and Brooks F (eds). *New Beginnings: Towards Patient and Public Involvement in Primary Care*. London: King's Fund, 2002.

13 Morris P and Trafford P. Learning from patients. In: Burton J and Jackson N (eds). *Work Based Learning in Primary Care*. Oxford: Radcliffe, 2004, pp. 87–102.

14 www.health-disciplines.ubc.ca/DHCC [accessed August 2006]. Published as Towle A and Weston W. Patient's voice in health professional education. *Patient Education and Counseling* 2006; **63**: 1–2.

15 www.leeds.ac.uk/medicine/men/voices06/index.html.

16 Whitehouse C, Morris P and Marks B. The role of actors in teaching medical communication. *Medical Education* 1984; **18**: 262–8.

17 Barrows H. *Simulated Patients: The Development and Use of a New Technique in Medical Education*. Springfield, Illinois: Charles C. Thomas, 1971.

18 Morris P. *The Development and Evaluation of Information-Giving and Health Education Skills for Medical Students and Doctors*. Cambridge: Health Promotion Research Trust, 1992.

19 Morris P, Armitage A, Symons J, Kilminster S, Roberts T, Dalton E, Muir D, Power S and Reed J. *Whose Voice is it Anyway: Embedding the Patient Voice in the Simulated and Standardized Patient*. Plenary paper presented at 'Where's the Patient Voice in Health Professional Education?' conference, Vancouver, 2005.

20 McNaughton N and Hodges B. *Where is the Patient in the Standardized Patient?* Paper presented at 'Where's the Patient Voice in Health Professional Education?' conference, Vancouver, 2005.

21 Association for the Study of Medical Education. *Lay Clinical Educators: Career Development and Accreditation*. www.asme.org.uk/conf_courses/2006/docs_pix/03_07_report.pdf. [accessed August 2006]. 7 March 2006.

22 Freire P. *Pedagogy of the Oppressed*. Harmondsworth: Penguin, 1972.

23 Bowlby J. *Attachment and Loss, Volume 1: Attachment*. London: Hogarth Press, 1969.

24 Scott Peck M. *The Road Less Travelled*. London: Arrow Books, 1978.

25 Dalton E and Morris P. Good communication: the patient perspective. *Medicine Newsletter*, November 2004. School of Medicine, University of Leeds.

26 Fresh Start courses run by the London Deanery GP department. www.londondeanery. ac.uk/gp/courses_conferences/pdf/Prospectus_2006_2007.pdf/.

27 Armitage A, O'Neill F, Morris P and Roberts T. The patient voice in medical education. *Clinical Teacher* (accepted).

28 Kilminster S, Hale C, Lascelles M, Morris P, Roberts T, Stark P, Sowter J and Thistlethwaite J. Learning from real life: patient-focused interprofessional workshops offer added value. *Medical Education* 2004; **38**: 717–26.

29 Thacker A, Perez W, Crabbe N, McCluskey C, Hollins S and Raji O. *The Contribution of Actors with Intellectual Disabilities to the Training of Medical Students*, 2006. On the intellectual disability section of the St George's Medical School website: www.intellectualdisability.info/how_to/actors_students.htm.

30 O'Neill F. *Developing a Strategic Approach to User and Carer Involvement in Pre-registration Nursing and Midwifery Education in Leeds*. Leeds: School of Healthcare Studies, 2002.

31 Gell C and Anderson J. *Learning with Users: Good Practice Guidelines*. Nottingham: mhhe, 2005.

32 A report of a meeting of GP educators on 14 March 2006, held by the London Deanery GP department. www.londondeanery.ac.uk/gp/primary_care_development/.

33 World Health Organization. *Preparing the Workforce for the 21st Century*. Geneva: WHO, 2005.

34 O'Neill F, Morris P and Symons J. Bridging the gap: learning with patient teachers in health professional education. *Practice Development in Health Care* 2006; **5** (1): 26–9 (www.interscience.wiley.com).

35 Pollock K. *Concordance in Medical Consultations: A Critical Review*. Oxford: Radcliffe, 2006.

36 Goldsmith J. *BMJ* 19 March 1999; **318**. eletters (bmj.bmjjournals.com).

37 Cayton H. Some thoughts on medical professionalism and regulation. *Defining and Developing Professionalism*. Association for the Study of Medical Education meeting, 28 April 2005. www.asme.org.uk/conf_courses/2005/docs_pix/04_28_cayton.pdf.

Electronic communication and issues relating to the consultation

David Topps

This chapter explores:

- email consultations • issues relating to the authentication of electronic data and communication • accessibility of doctors • internet • pervasive technology • lack of non-verbal communication • telehealth • legal issues • validity of information • doctor–computer communication.

SPOCK: 'Random chance seems to have operated
in our favour.'
McCOY: 'In plain, non-Vulcan English, we've been lucky.'
SPOCK: 'I believe I said that, Doctor.'

'THE DOOMSDAY MACHINE' · *Star Trek*

Box 10.1 ○ Glossary of terms used in this chapter

○ ***Ejaculation*** • sudden utterance or voluble expression.

○ ***Minute Muffler™*** • a chain of quick-fix automotive repair franchises in North America. 'While-U-Wait' etc.

○ ***Netiquette*** • internet etiquette. A few simple maxims in email and other internet correspondence.

○ ***SMS*** • Short Message System. For sending brief text messages by mobile phone: now commonly known as 'texting'.

○ ***Spam*** • unsolicited emails.

○ ***TLA*** • three letter abbreviations.

As clinicians head into the Information Age, the plethora of communication tools at their disposal increases daily. Doctors today may expect to communicate with patients using:

- telephone

- fax

- email

- mobile cellular phones or their SMS text

- pagers

- online discussion forums

- videoconferencing

as well as the traditional face-to-face and paper methods. However, will these tools be helpful in doctor–patient communications? They certainly present a new set of challenges. The anonymity of electronic media, speed of inter-action and limitless geography of the internet pose a variety of factors that both help and hinder effective interaction with patients.

Email consultations

A consultation, as previously defined, is a conference between two or more people to consider a particular question. Such a conference implies an exchange of views. Thus it is perfectly feasible within this definition to hold an email consultation. However, unlike telephone or face-to-face consulta-tions, email is hampered by the lag-time between each person's statement of views and posing of questions. It is possible to conduct internet conver-sations in real time, but what then is the advantage compared with more traditional interactions?

Email consultations are not interactive and it is therefore difficult to imag-ine their use by patients with acute or complex problems, where eliciting a history and the judicious use of questions are important. Examinations are of course impossible. A US study has shown that patients prefer telephone access and personal appointments to email communication, especially for complex or sensitive problems. However, those with internet access are happy to receive normal test results or advice about minor problems such as sore throats on-line.[1]

Patients who know their GP's email address have ease of access to per-sonal advice anywhere in the world. No longer may we feel relief when patient X disappears for a few months to the other side of the world. How-ever, this raises the question of whose responsibility is patient X if distant consultations are taking place? This is discussed later in the chapter. There is also the consideration of response time. Should a practice aim to deal with emails within a certain number of hours in the same way that other calls are dealt with? Certainly patients expect to receive a reply within 48 hours of their message.[2]

Car and Sheikh in the UK have conducted a systematic review of email consultations in health care and have come to the conclusion that successful communication in this medium depends on a clear and shared understanding by both doctor and patient of its role, advantages and limitations.[3] They suggest that GPs should initially consider developing a standard protocol to inform patients of the ways in which email communication will be used. This may include making appointments, patients feeding back information on blood glucose levels, obtaining test results, ordering repeat prescriptions and consultations for certain predefined problems.[4]

E-patients have been defined by Ferguson and Frydman of the USA as those who seek online guidance for their own health problems and the friends and relatives who go on-line on the patients' behalf.[5] The number of e-patients is likely to grow and therefore GPs must reflect on how they intend to interact with this breed of client.

Authentication

The faceless nature of electronic communications presents doctors with the challenge of knowing with whom they are communicating. How do they really know that the sender of that email message is the person purported? Email address spoofing is ridiculously simple and easy to disguise. And can the doctor, or the patient, really be sure that only the intended recipient will pick up the message on a voicemail system? A serious breach of confidentiality is quite easy to commit in such circumstances. The more serious and increasingly frequent problem of identity theft poses a greater threat so that the doctor cannot truly rely on the identity of the corresponding party, even with additional precautions. Because of this doubt, it is sensible to take a few basic precautions (Box 10.2).

A similar problem of authentication faces those who seek information from electronic sources such as the internet. There is a huge number of medically oriented websites but the ratio of wheat to chaff is poor.[6,7]

We'll address the challenge of information validity later in this chapter but, while we're discussing personal authentication, the challenge of personal credibility comes to the fore. The internet has given everyone the means to publish, so how can a patient judge if an author's credentials are worth the electronic certificate they are printed on? Anyone can be an expert. The global accessibility of such information means that patients can wander (and wonder) far afield in their quest, but impressively named

> **Box 10.2 ○ Steps to ensure confidentiality**
>
> ○ Avoid specifics, especially in touchy subject areas.
>
> ○ Stick to logistic information, like appointment availability.
>
> ○ Warn the patient that anything they write or say may go astray so they should also be careful.
>
> ○ Warn users of email systems that employers/owners have right of access.
>
> ○ Warn system users that they cannot assume confidentiality just because they are communicating with a doctor's office.
>
> ○ Avoid confirming information given by the patient – it may be speculative by another party.
>
> ○ Never write or say anything that you wouldn't be happy seeing printed on a newspaper front page.

colleges and organisations are no guarantee of studiousness and rigour. Even accrediting organisations now struggle with this issue: the Web has made it possible to buy a complete set of documents, certifying various forms of medical accomplishment, including a full degree. (See Chapter 4 for further discussion of evidence-based medicine.)

Doctors can help their patients to assess the credibility of such sources but they will be more convincing if they assume the role of sceptical adviser rather than cynical rejecter of unknown modalities.[8]

Accessibility

As well as increased accessibility of information, the information age promises us tools to enhance the accessibility of healthcare providers. We have rapidly progressed from telephone and postal communications (now affectionately known as snail mail) to a wide range of gadgets, all promising to make our lives easier. Doctors face a daily array of fax machines, pagers and voicemail systems, and are now also drowning in email, instant messaging and SMS interruptions. The well-connected doctor now risks looking like Batman with a utility belt of cacophonic appendages.

Yet, there is no denying the popularity of these communications tools. Current estimates suggest that over 595 million mobile phones will be sold over the next year[9] – a volume that shows no signs of abating (pun intended). To shun their use completely will be increasingly impractical; just hearken back to predictions made at the advent of the telephone.

This 'telephone' has too many shortcomings to be seriously considered as a means of communication. The device is inherently of no value to us.

WESTERN UNION *internal memo, 1876*

Ambivalence is common. We hate the intrusive warbler (a species that, sadly, is nowhere close to extinction) interrupting important meetings but woe betide the doctor who ignores the spousal plea for last-minute groceries on the drive home.

Which leads us to the question: will these multiple communications methods help us to communicate better? Will the doctor of tomorrow be more accessible? The automatic assumption that accessibility will improve may well be false. We risk plunging into a black hole of increasing electronic chaos as these multiple information streams converge and clash. Our brains are only hard-wired for three channels of concurrent communication: audio, visual and tactile/proprioceptive. Just try listening to two conversations at once to show how universal this is.

The business world has discarded the model of secretaries fending off unwanted invasions on executive time. Today's customers expect approachability and full-time availability. Is it inevitable that medicine will follow this road? While patients may enjoy such freedom of access, this may lead to inefficient use of precious resource time. Moreover, safety concerns abound when harried doctors conduct phone conversations while driving their cars, both activities vying for their attention – a scenario that is illegal in an increasing number of jurisdictions, including the UK.

So what can be done to prevent this deluge from engulfing the doctor? A few carefully selected strategies may ease the pressure (Box 10.3).

Does technology itself hold any promise in stemming the tide? It promises much but time will tell. All-in-one integrated devices that combine mobile phone, pager, wireless email and personal digital assistant show some promise for alleviating the Batman Belt Syndrome. True messaging integration, with intelligent electronic assistants that can field and redirect calls, according to priority and source, are some way off. Current attempts are laughable, not laudable ... but then Thomas Watson, Chief Executive at IBM, in 1943 scoffed at the world needing more than five computers.[10]

The internet

In all of this, our consumption of communications bandwidth is nearly as dramatic as our consumption of trees in the paper mills. In the developed

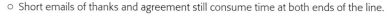
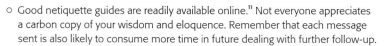

Box 10.3 ○ **Strategies to reduce communication overload**

○ Be selective in your communicating; just because it is easy to 'reach out and touch someone' does not mean that you should.

○ Leave your callback number at the beginning and end of a lengthy voicemail message. Replaying a monotonous monologue just to grab a misheard number is very frustrating.

○ Leave the times you expect to be available at that number. Endless rounds of telephone tag only please phone company accountants.

○ Use the appropriate medium; not everyone glances at their email daily; on the other hand, few of us like phone interruptions on non-urgent matters.

○ Short emails of thanks and agreement still consume time at both ends of the line.

○ Good netiquette guides are readily available online.[11] Not everyone appreciates a carbon copy of your wisdom and eloquence. Remember that each message sent is also likely to consume more time in future dealing with further follow-up.

○ Encourage others to follow these same suggestions: through your voicemail prompts, new patient handouts and clinical website advisories. If we all turn down the volume a little, we'll be able to hear each other.

world, we are now surprised when someone confesses to the lack of an email address. High-speed, full-time internet access is now commonplace in urban homes – a situation of which many a university would have been jealous merely one decade ago. But the ability to get on-line is not ubiquitous, even in the most affluent nations. Rural communities, as usual, are starved of these resources, despite having the greater need.[12]

The international situation is even worse. Developing nations do benefit from the Information Revolution. Some have been able to leapfrog the expense of installing an extensive landline system by going straight to wireless communications. However, sadly, the Digital Divide looks to be the widest and most rapidly expanding gap yet seen between the haves and the have-nots of this planet.[13]

There are simple measures that doctors may take to alleviate these trends. Apart from the steps suggested in Box 10.3, there are a few simple things that you can do to make life easier for those with low-speed connections (Box 10.4).

Pervasive technology

Like it or not, we are moving towards the world of ubiquitous computing.[14] A few years ago we scoffed at having an internet terminal on the refrigera-

Box 10.4 ○ Using email considerately

○ Use plain-text email when possible. HTML formatted emails are much larger.

○ Avoid large attachments such as photos, heavily formatted documents and sound recordings.

○ Be sparing when you quote the original message in your reply; don't be lazy and leave the whole thing in place when a few lines will suffice.

○ Be careful with auto-response messages like 'Away on vacation'; these can create a lot of clutter if two email systems start a ping-pong match between two absent parties.

○ Never reply to any spam, even to tell the senders to stop. It's just like voting – it only encourages them. Users of slow connections suffer much more from the effects of this scourge. Do your bit!

tor, yet many households find themselves leaving the computer connected all the time on making the move towards broadband internet access. It is now so easy to walk up to a terminal to find out when the movie is playing, watch our stocks bottom out or check our bank accounts that patients expect to be able to book a doctor's appointment on-line as well. This will no doubt be possible in a few years time. The concept of having access to information from anywhere at anytime has rapidly taken hold.

This cultural shift towards '24/7' availability is not solely related to the existence of the internet. We expect to do our grocery shopping on Sundays and late evenings. We have become accustomed to instant service, instant tellers, instant coffee, no matter the time of day. The Minute Muffler™ effect is affecting how we do business in every walk of life. Increasingly our patients also expect instant answers to their medical questions. If they can't see their own doctor at the time of their perceived crisis, they turn elsewhere for information and reassurance.

This can be a good thing. We have moved well beyond the paternalistic model described in Chapter 2 and welcome open discussion with our patient-centred approach and informed shared decision-making model. A well-informed consumer gets better value out of the healthcare system, is better motivated and has better outcomes overall. However, many a doctor has blanched at the sight of a six-inch stack of printouts, fresh from the internet, proudly produced by a persistent frequent attender. 'Will you just take a peek at these, doc?' This patient little realises that we don't even have time to keep up with the expected reading of the 4000+ medical journals that are currently in print let alone patient-recommended reading.[15] At this point, it can be useful to employ the services of your erstwhile literature-searcher a little further: 'It'll take me quite a few days to read through all the excellent stuff you've found and I'm concerned I may miss some key points if I rush. Why don't you take a first pass and highlight *no more than 4 key questions* that we can discuss at your appointment next week?' It is more important to address the questions that concern the patient than to digest fully the comprehensive load presented to you. An approach directed at the patient's concerns yields much more satisfaction than a skilfully crafted synopsis.

Just how pervasive should we allow the technology to be in the inner sanctum of the consulting room? A computer terminal is now commonplace, if not *de rigueur.* But how many doctors consider the positioning of the monitor screen? Traditional practice has promulgated secrecy in note taking, often unwittingly. We have tended to shroud the contents of our daily entries, to scrawl scripts illegibly or in Latin, and to use TLAs and jargon to excess. However, recent work in the study of medical error and systems failures has shown that patients are happier when they can see the screen and contribute to the accuracy of notes. Not only that – they are safer.[16, 17, 18]

The small size of personal digital assistants (PDAs) has sometimes been appreciated as being less intrusive in the confines of the office. Comfortably held on the lap, to me there is something intrinsically less irritating about writing on their little screens than the clatter of a keyboard. But these same little screens are harder to share between two or more people, thereby losing the advantage stated above – a co-pilot to watch your Palm Pilot™ data accuracy.

Non-verbal communication

As fully interacting human beings, we depend on more than words for communicating our thoughts and needs. It has been suggested that up to 93 per cent of our communication is non-verbal.[19] This oft-quoted proportion misrepresents the work of Albert Mehrabian, Professor of Psychology at MIT. The proportion varies significantly, according to the task at hand and the communications medium used. Nonetheless, the message is clear: we depend on more than words to be clear. This explains the increased tendency for electronic communications of all types to be misconstrued and applies particularly to messages with high emotional content. It is very unwise to conduct discussions that may become contentious or inflammatory in any way other than face to face. A new adage (if that's not oxymoronic) has developed: never send an email in anger; sleep on it or, at least, send it when calm.[20]

Since doctor–patient communications are much more likely to deal with delicate or contentious issues, these caveats should be heeded anew by any doctor who feels that the issues already raised in the preceding paragraphs have been successfully forestalled.

The absence of the more subtle clues of non-verbal communication and our marked dependence on them also appears to be one reason why video-conferencing has yet to meet its promise as a communications tool.[21] In the healthcare arena, it is widely used for educational and administrative purposes. However, when it comes to the more subtle process of doctor–patient communication, enthusiasm wanes quickly. Curiously, one exception to this seems to be telepsychiatry.

Telehealth

No discussion of doctor–patient communications and information technology can be complete without exploring telehealth. Telehealth refers to the use of communications technology, usually videoconferencing, for the purpose of enhancing the provision of health care. Indeed, for the past decade, the two would have been regarded by many as synonymous. Indicative of this would be that the *WONCA Policy Paper on Information Technology and Rural Health* focused entirely on this issue in its first edition and only broadened in scope when rewritten in 2002.[12]

As mentioned above, telehealth has fallen far short of its promises in most areas. Originally seen as a panacea to the manpower problems of rural health, centralist organisations zealously embraced and promoted its virtues. However, progress beyond well-publicised pilot projects has been slow in coming. Some of this is undoubtedly due to the limitations of the technology: low bandwidth, slow frame rates, poor resolution, and that most annoying effect of lag-time. This produces the slight delay in response that results in 'participant ping-pong', with each side over-talking the other. Perhaps our expectations were set too high by the early promulgators.

Beyond the technical, it is clear that other issues must be addressed for this technology to become widespread. Rural healthcare workers can be augmented but not replaced by centrally located expertise. Rural communities must be involved from the outset in planning and implementing these systems; a sense of ownership and involvement is essential to maintain not just the equipment but also the enthusiasm.[12]

The technical limitations can be overcome to some degree by sensible application of some simple steps. High-quality images take time to transmit over a slow connection but this does not preclude their use. This brings to mind the recent experience of a GP colleague involved in a teleradiology programme, grumbling about the 10 minutes that he had to wait for the images to download to his home, once he had slogged his way through the labyrinthine security processes of the hospital information system. When it was pointed out to him that this was likely the same time he would take to get dressed and back his car out of the garage, he wisely decided that this time could be profitably spent on fixing a midnight snack to accompany his perusal of the images. This *ad hoc* application of the store-and-forward principle illustrates something we can apply to many of our consults. 'Store-and-forward' refers to the process whereby images or other data are sent ahead for storage on a local computer before the need for them arises.

When saddled with a connection that is not adequate for full videoconferencing, it can be more profitable to focus on using the internet connection to share data, still images, files and written notes. There are several free programs such as MSN Messenger ™ or Yahoo IM ™ that facilitate online information sharing, instant messaging, white boarding and remote program operation, even over a very basic home setup. Audio communication is the most sensitive to lags and delays. It is not hard to establish a plain old telephone link to chat in the normal manner and without the attendant digital distortion and delays.

Of course, at the ongoing pace of technological development, this will be moot at some point in the future. How soon this happens is much less clear. It may be that one of the reasons that early promoters of videoconferencing were so bullish about its possibilities was that they expected all these hurdles to be brushed aside within a few years. There are, however, fascinating glimpses of what will be possible appearing on the event horizon of technology innovation – one just hopes that this is not the Hawking Radiation[22] produced by these technologies disappearing into their own black hole. As well as touch sensors and proprioceptive feedback loops exciting the surgeons with dreams of remote operating, there are even smell receptors available – which may not be an advantage for some of our patient interactions.

Legal issues

Telehealth has also brought with it some interesting legal challenges. Because the barriers of distance have essentially been removed, it is now technically quite feasible to hold consultations that cross many jurisdictional boundaries. Many groups are now wrestling with the issues of: whose patient is it anyway? Whose rules are we playing by? Simply applying the prior set of existing rules that govern one's own location is often shortsighted. And to avoid the issue by precluding such information exchange is not tenable in the long run – we live in an era of global information exchange and these pressures will not go away soon. It is naïve to expect that we will be able to adopt a uniform approach to such thorny problems. Common sense and forethought will be required, along with sensible flexibility – in which case, we'd better not leave it solely to the lawyers and politicians.

We are bound by the laws and rules currently in place, so it is sensible to clarify one's situation, if contemplating any kind of medical information exchange with a patient. Medical liability insurance companies are well aware of the pending issues, albeit less well able to give clear advice in all situations. However, it is worth seeking their opinion before electronic hell breaks loose. Many jurisdictions have already determined that money does not have to change hands, and physical presence does not have to have occurred in order to establish a doctor–patient relationship. Be careful.

Electronic communication has also brought another thorny legal issue to light: medical records. While most jurisdictions have clearly established that the patient has an intrinsic right to know their medical information, responsibility for maintaining the integrity, continuity, accuracy and privacy of the medical record is becoming more complex to define. It is axiomatic in most areas that the originator of the information is responsible for its accuracy and adequate longevity. This is simple when we are looking at systems that operate in isolation but, as we move inexorably towards complexly shared information, these boundaries become much more blurred. Take, for example, a lab order transmitted for a PSA test, along with the age and date of birth of the patient. Suppose further that the age and date of birth do not correspond. The lab sends back a result, along with a normal range that is dependent on the age given for the patient. Whose responsibility is it when the result is wrongly flagged as being out of range? Which system should be checking which information? This particular example is not that hard to sort out but the process of increasingly shared medical databases will make this more complex and commonplace.

Shared information brings many potential advantages. Reduction of medical error has already been demonstrated by the use of centrally stored databases of allergies and current medications. Further benefits can be had by the use of master problem lists and laboratory results. However, how much of this information should be shared and who with? As advocates for our patients, it behoves us to advise them appropriately on the risks of excessive disclosure or withholding of pertinent information. This will sometimes be a fine line to tread – not something that can be addressed with global release of information pro formas. Where such information is to be stored raises other tricky issues. Is it better to trust a central repository, safe behind Fort Knox-like security but possibly under government control? Or is it better to place one's faith in the server of the trusty local GP, whose server might well be below the radar horizon of central government but is wide open to the ministrations of her teenage hacker son.

Validity of information

With internally generated medical information, the responsibility for accuracy and validity of the information lies with the originator, as previously mentioned. But what about the information available from more general sources? Both as information 'reseller' and as patient advocate, doctors have a role to guide their patients on the path towards becoming as well informed as possible on health-related issues. Patients are increasingly turning to a broad variety of sources for their medical information: their herbalist, hypnotist and hairdresser all happily venture an opinion on what ails them. These erstwhile advisers are not bound by the niceties of evidence-based practice, a principle that is also losing devotees in mainstream medicine for its lack of individualisation of advice. Doctors will have to become adept at sifting the wheat from the chaff, while maintaining a respectful and respected relationship with their patients. The plethora of well-meaning, ill-informed but voluble internet discussion groups threatens to drown out civilised, thoughtful discussion. Media sensationalism, in the pursuit of readers and viewers, has dramatised the most innocuous of medical reports. Increasingly, one hears the phrase 'studies suggest that' followed by frenzied commentary that evokes the imminent collapse of the heavens. Keeping abreast of the latest implant scare or premature ejaculations of a researcher whose trial has ended early is increasingly difficult but our patients continue to trust our wise guidance.[23,24,25]

Augmenting the consultation

With so much information freely available on the internet, the concept of the value of information is sometimes hard to convey to patients. This appears more marked in services where the apparent cost of health care is more hidden. Ringing patients back who have requested advice calls is standard practice in the UK. At one time many practices insisted on returning calls on landlines due to the added expense of mobile phone calls. However, for many patients now their only phone is mobile. GPs have absorbed the extra costs. In health services where patients are charged for consultations, e.g. Australia, the USA and Canada, the problem of payment for telephone consultations is more difficult to overcome. In these countries doctors often freely, in the financial sense, converse by phone with clients whereas solicitors bill by the minute. Not that we want to stoop to such reconciling of the hours but the issue will become more poignant as teleconsulting and other forms of remote information exchange become more common.

However, we should not forget that we are information vendors in the Information Age, which by nature means that there is some inherent competition. Those who idle along in the slow lane of the information highway risk being run off into the ditch by speeding data peddlers or, at least, bypassed in the past. What can we do to bolster our sagging credibility index? Use those tools that threaten to engulf us. Rather than sheepishly proffering tattered old patient handout sheets, with outdated data and risible recommendations, the clinical information systems (electronic medical records systems) now in development offer the capability of individualised advice. These go far beyond the tired approach of lottery-style 'Dear Householder' salutations – their talk, tips and titbits are tailored to the demographics, demeanour and diet of that person. Pulling such information directly from the patient record, these systems hold the promise that future customisation may include allowances for body surface area, hepatic, renal and cognitive function so that the right medication in the right dose and container is dispensed, along with the right warnings, advice and lifestyle admonishments. Recalls for preventive maintenance or result follow-up can be appropriately targeted, with a pre-distributed preface that can make the next consultation more effective for all parties.

Doctor–computer communication

Unless we follow the predictions of Ray Kurzweil, a leading pundit on artificial intelligence, sooner than he anticipated,[26] and start having cybernetically augmented patients to look after, this section is not about treating the dastardly devices but about more effective means of communicating all that precious information from the doctor to the disk. Many a doctor has been heard to say 'what on hers argue stalking about?' – no, seriously – many appear to be waiting for that holy grail of accurate voice recognition before they will take seriously the notion of interacting extensively with a computerised system. Voice recognition has improved enormously over the past few years and currently compares with a dyslexic child in its accuracy for anything other than sustained, predictable dictation. For short notes, which lack the surrounding contextual information, it is still amusing to see what is generated with one's utterances.

There is some hope with systems that are designed around template-driven voice recognition. Imagine a form where, for each box, there is only a limited set of possible entries. For example, you make a diagnosis of cystitis and dictate this to the computer. The computer then has a much easier time picking from a word list of a dozen antibiotic names, than from the entire 60,000 word vocabulary. However, talking to a computer is highly intrusive on doctor–patient communications – if you don't believe me, just try talking to a simple Dictaphone *during* your next consultation. As mentioned earlier, our brains are limited in their communications channels. Doctors can easily read from a screen or type on a keyboard while listening to a patient, not that one would be rude enough to do it all the time, as some overlapping multitasking is socially quite permissible. Patients are used to computers in consultations and do not consider that such technology affects the doctor–patient relationship.[27] But start talking to your electronic medical record system and the patient instantly clams up.

The ideal electronic system should allow the GP to record the patient's story or narrative with minimum effort and the ability to add sketches as well as speech at the surgery desk (and even the bedside).[28] Of course, in the future, it is possible that we could have full-time, real-time recording of the consultation, like flight recorders on aircraft. In fact, recent comparisons of the woeful state of the medical industry, and its accident rate, with the stellar safety record of the airline industry make such possibilities far from remote. The advantage would be that the smart computer system would interpret your conversation flow and, like Radar O'Reilly from the television series *MASH*, presciently offer information on its screens. The disadvantage

---

Use of technology by patients ○ *reflections*

I guess the cartoon of a troublesome patient with yards of info printed off the net is out of date now really, as more GPs become comfortable with surfing the net themselves. But the fear of being flooded with demands and expectations is still with us. As always, GPs coming clean about the limits of their knowledge and feeling comfortable doing so seems to be the key. Some GPs I work with say they feel happy seeing such patients as co-researchers and, as such, give them guidance about critical reading and good sites. Patients in our educational and research groups say the growing use of blogs by patients as a therapeutic tool is helpful – as are those by health workers. Some patients can only communicate with each other about their patient experience electronically – those who are isolated or with infection issues. We encourage the use of electronic communication by students in health care, who are most comfortable with it. Perhaps the new conversations we need between patients and patients, and between patients, students and professionals, will be helped by all these new, and therefore perturbing, devices.

Computers in the consulting room ○ *reflections*

Where would we be without the desktop computer? Within a relatively few years these machines have become almost as necessary as the stethoscope. The paperless practice is a reality (though there still seems to be a lot of written documents flying around). My next step is to involve the computer more for the obvious benefit of the patient, rather than as a systems tool. I need to make better use of patient information on the internet, decision aids and better diagrams than my poor pencil outlines. However, I also need to reduce the obtrusiveness of the VDU in the doctor–patient interaction at certain points of the consultation. How often do I address that screen rather than the patient? We make an uneasy threesome sometimes. Certainly email consultations suffer from lack of non-verbal cues, but so do face-to-screen consultations when the patient is left staring at my right ear while I clatter away with the keyboard.

---

is that every word would be taken down and could be used against you – I can just see the lawyers rubbing their hands with glee.

○ Summary

- Email consultations are likely to become more common as patients realise their value. However, such consultations are not interactive and it is therefore difficult to imagine their use by patients with acute or complex problems.

- GPs should initially consider developing a standard protocol to inform patients of the ways in which email communication will be used.

- Confidentiality is a major issue with electronic communication, as is the absence of non-verbal communication.

- A well-informed patient gets better value out of the healthcare system, is better motivated and has better outcomes overall, so GPs therefore need to welcome their patients' use of the internet as an aid to shared information.

- GPs have a role as validators of internet information.

REFERENCES

1 Katz S J, Moyer C A, Cox D T and Stern D T. Effect of a triage-based e-mail system on clinic resource use and patient and physician satisfaction in primary care. A randomized controlled trial. *Journal of General Internal Medicine* 2003; **18**: 736–44.

2 Couchman G R, Forjuoh S N and Rascoe T G. E-mail communications in family practice: what do patients expect? *Journal of Family Practice* 2001; **50**: 414–18.

3 Car J and Sheikh A. Email consultations in health care: 1 – scope and effectiveness. *BMJ* 2004; **329**: 435–8.

4 Car J and Sheikh A. Email consultations in health care: 2 – acceptability and safe application. *BMJ* 2004; **329**: 439–42.

5 Ferguson T and Frydman G. The first generation of e-patients. *BMJ* 2004; **328**: 1148–9.

6 Eysenbach G and Kohler C. How do consumers search for and appraise health information on the World Wide Web? Qualitative study using focus groups, usability tests, and in-depth interviews. *BMJ* 2002; **324**: 573–7.

7 Health on the Net (HON) Foundation Survey: Evolution of Internet use for health purposes 2001. www.hon.ch/Survey/FebMar2001/survey.html [accessed August 2006].

8 Cochrane JD. Healthcare @ the speed of thought. *Integrated Healthcare Report* 1999; **1–14**: 16–17.

9 IDC Report quoted by Cellular News. www.cellular.co.za/news_2004/june/062404-phone-shipments-1q04.htm [accessed August 2006].

10 Rinaldi AH. User Guidelines and Netiquette. www.cs.biu.ac.il/home/leagal/netguide [accessed August 2006].

11 Amusing Quotes. www.amusingquotes.com/h/1/439.htm [accessed August 2006].

12 Topps D, Togno J, Strasser R, Hovel J and Wynn-Jones J. *WONCA Policy Paper on Information Technology and Rural Health.* Second edition. 2002. www.globalfamilydoctor.com/aboutWonca/working_groups/write/itpolicy/ITPoli.htm [accessed August 2006].

13 Smith R. Closing the digital divide. *BMJ* 2003; **326**: 238.

14 Weiser M. *Ubiquitous Computing.* 1996. www.ubiq.com/hypertext/weiser/UbiHome.html [accessed August 2006].

15 Haynes R B, McKibbon K A, Fitzgerald D, Guyatt G H, Walker C J and Sackett D L. How to keep up with the medical literature: III. Expanding the number of journals you read regularly. *Annals of Internal Medicine* 1986; **105**: 474–8.

16 Als A B. The desktop computer as a magic box: patterns of behaviour connected with the desktop computer; GPs' and patients' perceptions. *Family Practice* 1997; **14**: 17–23.

17 Ridsdale L and Hudd S. Computers in the consultation: the patient's view. *BJGP* 1994; **44**: 367–9.

18 Makoul G, Curry R H and Tang P C. The use of electronic medical records: communication patterns in outpatient encounters. *Journal of the American Medical Informatics Association* 2001; **8**: 610–15.

19 Mehrabian A. *Silent Messages: Implicit Communication of Emotions and Attitudes*. Belmont, CA: Wadsworth, 1990.

20 Group IT. *Mailing List Guidelines*. 2001. www.infodiv.unimelb.edu.au/email/student/etiquette.html [accessed August 2006].

21 Yellowlees P. An analysis of why telehealth systems in Australia have not always succeeded. *Journal of Telemedicine and Telecare* 2001; **7 (Suppl. 2)**: 29–31.

22 Hawking S W. *A Brief History of Time*. New York: Bantam, 1998.

23 Blake J M, Collins J A, Reid R L, Fedorkow D M, Lalonde A B, Christilaw J, Fortier M, Fortin C, Jolly E E, Lemay A, O'Grady T, Smith T E, Cooper J, Maxted J M, O'Grady K and Turek M A. The SOGC statement on the WHI report on estrogen and progestin use in postmenopausal women. *Journal of Obstetrics and Gynaecology Canada* 2002; **24**: 783–90, 793–802.

24 Passalacqua R, Campione F, Caminiti C, Salvagni S, Barilli A, Bella M, Barni S, Barsanti G, Caffo O, Carlini P, Cinquemani G, Di Costanzo F, Giustini L, Labianca R, Mazzei A, Olmeo N, Paccagnella A and Toscano L. Patients' opinions, feelings, and attitudes after a campaign to promote the Di Bella therapy. *Lancet* 1999; **353**: 1310–14.

25 Passalacqua R, Caminiti C, Salvagni S, Barni S, Beretta G D, Carlini P, Contu A, Di Costanzo F, Toscano L and Campione F. Effects of media information on cancer patients' opinions, feelings, decision-making process and physician–patient communication. *Cancer* 2004; **100**: 1077–84.

26 Kurzweil R. *The Age of Spiritual Machines: When Computers Exceed Human Intelligence*. New York: Penguin Putnam, 2000.

27 Solomon G L. Are patients pleased with computer use in the examination room? *Journal of Family Practice* 1995; **41**: 241–4.

28 Walsh S H. The clinician's perspective on electronic health records and how they affect patient care. *BMJ* 2004; **328**: 1184–7.

The consultation in the 21st century

This chapter recaps the summary material already presented and provides a template for the 21st-century consultation. This template summarises the evidence and refers to relevant chapters, rather than repeating the primary references. New material includes advice on conducting telephone consultations and recording consultations. There is a number of issues for discussion; we certainly do not have the answers to all the dilemmas facing today's GPs.

Before the consultation

The following are factors that affect the quality of consultations – issues to be considered by GPs and their practices.

- Continuity of care is still important but not always necessary, and not of equal importance for every consultation.

- Patients prefer their personal doctor or regular GP for complex problems. This has implications for access and appointment systems.

- There must be good communication between team members if continuity is not always possible and because patients will see various members of the primary healthcare team for different problems and activities. The practice must ensure good record keeping and define access to records to ensure team continuity while respecting confidentiality.

- Minimum consultation length as a marker of quality and improved outcome is 10 minutes but in reality this is too short for many consultations. Consultation length within the present healthcare system needs to be discussed. Is there a system in the practice for offering patients longer consultations if necessary?

Choice of doctor: the patient's perspective

- With many GPs choosing to work part time or because of other working commitments, patients may not be able to see the doctor of their choice. Advanced access also means that doctor choice is limited on certain days. The effects this has on the doctor–patient relationship and GPs' way of working are not clear. Patients who are used to seeing their 'own' doctor may feel disgruntled. Patients who are used to seeing a different doctor on every occasion will be less unsettled.

- Patients should be allowed the choice of seeing a 'new' doctor if they wish. They may have something they wish to talk about without complications arising from their past encounters. The 'new' doctor should try to explore ideas, concerns and expectations but not probe too deeply if the patient makes it clear that this is not needed during the present consultation.

- However, 'frequent attenders' should be encouraged to see the same doctor. This may indeed be part of their agreed management plan.

- Patients with complex management issues should be managed by one doctor if possible, or a team approach adopted with good communication and record keeping. This is particularly important for patients who are drug misusers, drug dependent or liable to 'use the system' to obtain what they want.

- Patients who deliberately choose to see another doctor for a second or even third opinion cannot be stopped from doing this in any practical sense. It is up to the doctor to spot what is going on and to explore the reasons for this with the patient. However, our modern way of working means that patients cannot be blamed for the loss of continuity and their making use of this modern system to 'shop around'.

- GPs must be careful to ensure the suitability and credentials of locums working within their practices. Locum doctors must be on a Primary Care Organisation list but their indemnity and qualifications should also be checked before they start work. They should be identified to patients as locums and the length of time they will be in the practice stated. This may affect a patient's choice of doctor seen.

- Patients should also be aware of the status of GP registrars. They should also be informed when booking an appointment of any plans for a medical student or other health professional sitting in with the doctor and given the opportunity to decline to see the doctor under those circumstances.

Seeing the nurse first?

- When patients attend the emergency department or out-patient clinic, their vital signs are usually assessed by a health professional before they see the doctor. This may include height, weight, pulse, blood pressure, temperature and blood sugar level if relevant. Such measurements are rarely carried out in primary care unless the patient is attending a special clinic such as for diabetes or ischaemic heart disease. Should patients in general practice consult with a practice nurse first for health promotion purposes? Would it be helpful for doctors if these results were available, or would they divert the doctor from the patient's underlying problems? Would they deflect the patient from their concern and upset the rehearsed introductory comments?

- A blood pressure reading may be useful but a high figure made known to the patient may cause enough anxiety to deflect them from their own agenda. What is the role of health promotion activities in the routine consultation?

The consultation itself

Introductions

- As appropriate; these include the position of the doctor in the practice and whether they are permanent, short term or a locum GP. Never assume the patient knows who you are and your position in the practice, unless this is a regular patient of yours. Whether the doctor is going to be available in the future may affect the patient's presentation of the problem or story.

- Whether GP registrars should explain their status in the practice at this stage is open to debate. The practice leaflet should inform patients of the status of a practice as a training practice and what this entails.

- Patients should also be aware of the level of pre-registration house officers (foundation year 1 doctors) and their need to have prescriptions signed by their supervisor. It is best to be up-front with these issues to avoid complications.

- It is also important to introduce anyone else who is present in the consulting room and the reason for their presence. For example, there may be a medical student or GP registrar sitting in. Best practice is to advise the patient of this prior to the consultation. The receptionist should ask for consent when booking in the patient but the doctor must check that the patient is happy at the beginning of the consultation. Written consent is also needed for videotaping of consultations at the beginning and end of the encounter.

- Any person accompanying the patient should be identified. Is this a family member, carer, interpreter, advocate or friend? What is this person's role in the consultation? Teenage girls often consult with the support of a friend or their mother. It is best not to assume the relationship but to ask if no introduction is forthcoming.

- While it may be assumed that the patient is happy for the accompanying person to be present in the consultation, this should also be ascertained. A young patient may wish to be offered the chance to talk to the doctor by himself or herself for part or all of the consultation.

Opening remarks

- An ongoing doctor–patient relationship of months to years may start in different ways. Perhaps it starts with an opening few remarks on either side regarding family or social matters. If the doctor has written a note that the patient was about to go on holiday after the last consultation, a question about the holiday may be a pleasant way to start proceedings. However, this runs the risk of deflecting the patient from the problem, particularly if it is new, or the holiday may have been disastrous, leaving the patient with the decision of how much to say.

- Similarly if the doctor has been away the patient may mention this and ask about the 'holiday'. If the doctor's absence was other than happy, it is probably best not to answer in too much detail.

- Patients may expect a new doctor to be familiar with their story because of the records or discussion in the practice. The doctor may choose to start by saying that they have not met before and invite the patient to start the story from the beginning, even though there are notes from previous encounters.

Presentation and exploration of patient's problems

- This exploration includes: the medical and psychosocial history; the patient's ideas, concerns and expectations; identification of wants and needs; and relevant past medical history. It draws on both the patient's narrative and questions by the doctor. If this part of the consultation goes badly it is difficult to recover and gain a good outcome.

- We want a focused history in order to make a diagnosis; the focus depends on the doctor and patient. The biopsychosocial, patient-centred and narrative approaches help ensure that the focus is not too narrow.

- Interruptions from phone calls, distractions from the computer and holdovers from previous consultations are not conducive to good consultation skills. Each doctor needs to give instructions to reception and other staff as to which telephone calls need to be answered and which may wait until between patients.

- Obviously the patient's first volunteered reason for attendance may not be the most important or sole problem. The key skill here is listening with judicious use of open and closed questions as appropriate. Empathy is important.

- However, you should not assume that there is always a hidden agenda. Some patients' problems are simple and are exactly as the patient describes them.

- In a follow-up consultation it is important to find out if the patient has new issues to discuss. This is rather than assuming that it is simply a matter of seeing if the previous problems have been resolved or if the condition is stable, or to monitor ongoing problems as relevant.

- If a patient presents with a list of problems and these are not all interrelated, doctor and patient need to negotiate which problems should be dealt with at this consultation and which may be left until the next.

Physical examination as necessary

- As this book concentrates on communication within the consultation there has been no discussion about issues arising from examination. Many consultations do not include any physical examination at all. Some have touch; for example, when a patient is distressed the doctor may hold the patient's hand. Allow ample time for the patient to undress and ideally the patient should be left to do this unless assistance is needed. The patient should also be given time to dress without feeling rushed, whatever strain this places on the doctor to keep to time.

- The consultation moves into another stage once there is contact. The reason for an examination must be given, especially examinations that involve the removal of clothing and those of an intimate nature.

- The doctor and patient should decide if a chaperone is necessary. The information sharing may continue during the examination, and if a third party is present this must be acknowledged, consent obtained from the patient and the presence of this person documented in the notes. The NHS Clinical Governance Support Team has published a model chaperone framework. It states: 'For most patients respect, explanation, consent and privacy take precedence over the need for a chaperone. The presence of a

third party does not negate the need for adequate explanation and cour-
tesy and cannot provide full assurance that the procedure or examination
is conducted appropriately.'[1]

- It is best not to give too much information in the course of the examination, as an embarrassed patient will not remember it. Starting a discussion
  on management with a semi-naked patient is not good practice. The doctor
  should say 'I will explain what I have found once you are dressed and sitting down again.'

Doctor and patient consider the nature and cause of the problem(s)

- If the patient presents with a list of problems and issues to discuss, the
  doctor may need to negotiate with the patient what should be covered in
  this consultation. There will be a need to prioritise the problems.

- This involves identifying physical, psychological and social factors as necessary: the biopsychosocial approach.

- If the doctor has explored the patient's ideas and concerns they will know
  if the possible diagnoses will be a surprise or otherwise to the patient.

- There may be some disagreement as to the cause of the problem if the
  patient's health beliefs have not been explored and information shared
  about opinions on both sides.

- The patient may wish to discuss material found on the internet. If this
  comprises a lot of material, the doctor may need to advise that this cannot
  be read at this time and decide whether it is necessary to peruse this at a
  later time.

- For chronic conditions and/or follow-up consultations this step also needs
  to be taken, the doctor checking the understanding of the patient, especially if this doctor has not consulted with this patient before. It is easy
  to assume that information has been shared on prior occasions, or that it
  has been remembered.

Doctor and patient consider the patient's health as a whole (holistic approach)

- This stage includes exploration of other possible contributing factors and
  concurrent problems.

- An important consideration in any consultation is how much opportunistic health promotion should be included. This will depend of course on the nature of the patient's problem and any reaction to shared information. Certain actions may be insensitive in this consultation but important for the patient's overall health status. For example a patient coming in to discuss a bereavement and difficulties coping may not wish to be reminded that she has not had a cervical smear for 10 years. A middle-aged man who has been made redundant may not feel it is important to have his blood pressure measured.

- The doctor's experience, intuition and philosophy all have a part to play in deciding how to proceed.

- If the patient has been seen and assessed by a nurse prior to the consultation, this is the point at which to discuss any abnormal physical findings if not mentioned before.

- Discussing health promotion and disease prevention may not be feasible if consultation time is running short. The GP needs to decide what to do if there are issues that do need to be discussed at some time, now or in the future. Will this patient return if the reason to come again is not directly related to the presenting problem?

Management by negotiation

- The doctor discusses possible treatment or management options, asks the patient about any other options they have read about or wish to discuss, outlines possible sequelae of the patient's condition and the benefits and risks of these possible management plans, drawing on an evidence-based approach and the doctor's own experience, and taking into account the patient's expectations as previously elicited.

- The doctor acknowledges if the patient does not want to be involved in decision making but finds this out from the patient rather than making a value judgement about the patient's wish to be involved.

- The doctor is careful not to introduce bias on the basis of his or her own preferred plan, but needs to take into account the cost-effectiveness of treatments and any current legal issues: informed shared decision making.

- The doctor needs to ask for the patient's opinion on the suggested management options and find out if the patient has expectations that will not be met by these strategies.

- The patient may need time to consider the options and may wish to have material to read or watch to help in this decision-making process.

- A decision aid may be helpful if the patient has access to the internet and a suitable aid is available for the particular problem/dilemma. The doctor needs to be aware of the content of the aid before recommending it.

Doctor and patient agree together on the plan

- The doctor checks that the patient has understood what has taken place in the consultation and the chosen management plan.

- The doctor asks the patient if there are any further questions or concerns.

- The doctor arranges with the patient a suitable follow-up strategy. Follow-up is an important part of the process, as the patient and doctor need to be clear about what is to happen next. These arrangements should be noted in the records. In some practices the doctor may make the appointment for the patient. In time this may also apply to hospital appointments.

- If a referral to secondary care or an outside agency is to be made, the patient should be informed about how long it is likely to be before an acknowledgement letter or date is received.

- If the patient is to have investigations or blood tests, they need to know about arrangements for receiving the results. This is all information sharing but it is sometimes forgotten in the end stage of the consultation. Writing down such information for patients is helpful.

- The doctor and patient may wish to discuss whether any part of the follow-up procedure is possible by email and, if so, the arrangements for this need to be outlined.

Finishing off

- The doctor checks the patient's understanding and that both the doctor and patient know what is to happen next.

- The doctor invites further questions or comments.

- If the consultation is running over time the doctor should acknowledge this. Some of the tasks of this consultation may be able to be deferred until another time.

After the consultation

Medical records

- Make good notes. (Consider making these with the patient present.)

- While a lot has been written about patient access to records and computerised or electronic records and their contents over the last few years, little has been discussed about what a doctor should actually write as a permanent record of a consultation. True, we are exhorted by the defence bodies to make full contemporaneous notes that may be used as evidence if necessary. We have also been advised not to put offensive remarks in writing, unlike our predecessors who had little fear of their patients seeing their true opinions.

- In *Good Medical Practice* the General Medical Council stipulates that doctors 'must keep clear, accurate and contemporaneous patient records that report the relevant findings, decisions made, information given to patients and any drugs or treatment prescribed'.[2]

- Making a true record of a 10-minute consultation is an art. The notes need to be easy to understand, give the kernel of the problem and what is going to happen, be intelligible to colleagues (and ideally to patients) and be written in the short time between patients. They are important to ensure continuity of care.

- Questions arise as to this process. Should the doctor write notes while listening to the patient? This obviously reduces the amount of eye contact but possibly gives the patient the sense that the doctor is listening as dictation proceeds. Should the doctor write the notes while they summarise what the patient has said? A complicated history is often difficult to remember once the patient leaves the room. Adding to it later if further facts are remembered may appear to be an attempt to cover up omissions. Indeed, certain computer programmes do not allow additions to be made to consultation records once the record has been closed, or certainly not the next day.

- With the move to shared decision making the doctor needs to decide how much of the discussion of options, negotiation and compromise needs to be recorded. There are no easy answers to these questions.

- The move to computerisation has encouraged minimal note keeping.[3] Not surprisingly doctors are liable to miss recording home visits electronically, though some doctors now take hand-held computers or laptops on visits.

Hand-written notes at the time of the visit may be transferred later to the computerised records and doctors are then less likely to miss recording important details. Within consultations doctors appear to record fewer symptoms and write less about their severity on computer compared with paper records. This may be due partly to the programmes used and the keyboard skills of doctors, and therefore an improvement in electronic record keeping should occur over time as technology makes note recording easier. However, the doctor still needs to think about quality and quantity. What should be summarised about this interaction?

- Chapter 10 includes more about electronic medical records.

- If a doctor decides to continue to keep paper records these should be dated and legible.

Personal development plans (PDPs)

- As an educational activity, record the consultation for PDP/appraisal purposes, with a reflective element. A description of a consultation does not indicate what the doctor has learned from the encounter. During the consultation the doctor may realise that they have a learning need and this may be written in the learning plan of the PDP, with details of how the learning need will be met, and, later, with evidence that it has been met. This process requires reflection. One example of how this might be done is through the PUNs and DENs process as devised by Dr Richard Eve, a British GP. PUN is a patient's unmet need and DEN is a doctor's educational needs.[4]

- Chapter 8 provides information about the means of assessing consultation skills. Revalidation and appraisal include a doctor providing evidence of competence in practice. This evidence will usually be collected as a portfolio. The PDP is a tool that, together with the portfolio and an activity log, provides a record of personal learning.

- A PDP includes educational priorities, usually for a year, which a doctor has decided are important in the context of their practice and learning needs. These priorities will of course vary from GP to GP and may consist of areas such as clinical topics (e.g. new drugs for diabetes), management issues (e.g. health and safety at work legislation) and new skills (e.g. insertion of contraceptive implants).

- Some doctors will also want to focus on consulting skills. Perhaps they have a problem with frequent attenders or patients with unexplained symptoms, or they lack confidence in breaking bad news or dealing with aggressive people. Lack of skill in a particular area of a consultation may be apparent from something that 'goes wrong': did a patient burst into tears because of something I said? Did a patient storm out of the consulting room because I refused to issue a certificate? Did I feel uncomfortable when dealing with a bereaved husband? Did I become angry with a patient who had not taken his medication properly? These critical incidents may be analysed and reflected upon. These sorts of questions facilitate reflection. Perhaps the incident happened because I was tired. I may have been distracted by the thoughts of another consultation or worried about a situation at home. Or I may simply need to refresh or improve my consulting behaviour.

● Chapters 7 and 9 explore ways in which groups of GPs may enhance their understanding and performance of the consultation. Video, peer review and work with simulated patients (SPs) are methods that may be helpful.

● In the broad area of consultation skills the PDP should focus on more specific issues. Rughani has identified eight questions to be answered when setting an educational priority (Box 11.1)[5] and these may be used to help plan learning and to consider what evidence is required for the portfolio.

● The objectives will include an element of improving skills so evidence needs to be collected that shows such improvement has occurred. Depending on the particular skills under scrutiny, rating of videotapes of consultations may be required, the rating being done both by self and a colleague or medical educator. However, the other methods listed in Chapter 8 may be considered. Reflection on consultations is also an important component of this.

Box 11.1 ○ Questions for PDPs[5]

○ What is the general area in which I need to learn?

○ How have I established this need?

○ What is the aim of my learning?

○ What are the specific objectives that I wish to achieve?

○ How do I intend to achieve these objectives?

○ How will I evaluate my development plan?

○ How will I demonstrate that I have undertaken this plan?

○ What is my timescale?

Telephone consultations

How do telephone consultations differ from the face-to-face meetings discussed so far? There is an assumption that communications skills are easily transferred to these types of interactions. Training is rarely given. Some of the issues are discussed in Chapter 10.

Patients ring for advice calls. Doctors offer advice on the telephone rather than make a house call or offer a patient an appointment. Investigation results are commonly given out this way. Telephone consultations are usually convenient for both parties but in certain situations may generate anxiety in either party. There is an obvious lack of detail from body language and non-verbal communication. Doctors worry about missing serious conditions without the opportunity to assess the patient's appearance.[6] In spite of the relative importance of the history, without the potential to carry out even the most minimal of examinations doctors are wary of diagnoses based on the patient's story alone.[7] It is difficult to adopt a patient-centred approach at a distance, and telephone consultations should be reserved for mild acute problems, simple questions that patients have or to check that treatment is going to plan once the patient has been thoroughly assessed at least once face to face. However, the introduction of such services as NHS Direct in the UK has demonstrated to patients that medical advice may be given by telephone in certain circumstances. Ringing one's own general practice means that such advice may be available from a familiar GP rather than an anonymous respondent.

Most practices have offered telephone consultations for many years. Patients are called back usually after morning surgery. Some practices have a system of a half-an-hour telephone spot each morning specifically to speak to patients who ring in.

Protocol for telephone consultations is similar to that for surgery consultations. The content and process should be considered (Box 11.2). Car (a PhD student in patient–doctor partnership in London) and Sheikh (a national primary care postdoctoral fellow in London) have suggested that an adequate telephone consultation for a specified problem should be of comparable length to a face-to-face interaction for the same problem.[8] This means that such consultations would not save time for doctors unless they took place instead of home visits. However, they would save time for patients.

To assess the quality of telephone consultations audiotaping is possible, with the consent of the patient. How often do we record our phone consultations for educational purposes and submit these to the same type of reflection that we use for videotaping?

Box 11.2 ○ Telephone consultations

Content of telephone consultations

○ When initiating or answering the phone call give name and designation.

○ Ensure that the correct patient is on the line and check the number.

○ Try to speak to the patient directly. If this is not possible ensure that the relationship of the patient to the caller is known.

○ Elicit the history and summarise.

○ Explore the patient's expectation of the call and what is needed.

○ Provide advice if appropriate or suggest that an appointment is made.

○ Ask the patient to repeat what has been said to check understanding.

○ Arrange follow-up.

○ Record the patient's name, time of call, length of call and content of call.

○ If possible the patient should disconnect first.

Process

○ Listening is important but ensure the patient knows you are still on the line.

○ Be alert for verbal cues such as lowering of voice, hesitations and signs of distress.

○ Allow pauses but remember the patient may worry about disconnection.

○ Invite the patient to ask questions.

Conclusion

General practitioners, other members of the primary healthcare team and health professionals should be constantly aware of the quality of their consultations and the framework of the practice within which they offer such consultations to patients. Communication and consultation skills atrophy if they are not reviewed. GPs are faced each day with complex and disturbing interactions. They need to update their strategies and skills just as they keep up-to-date with their clinical knowledge. A consultation is a big event in the lives of many patients and is hopefully a satisfying experience for most, even if the doctor is not able entirely to satisfy a patient's needs. Good communication, sharing information and involving patients in decisions about their own health is good practice.

REFERENCES

1 www.cgsupport.nhs.uk/Primary_Care/Resources.asp#chaperone_framework [accessed August 2006].

2 General Medical Council. *Good Medical Practice*. London: GMC, 2001.

3 Hamilton W T, Round A P, Sharp D and Peters T J. The quality of record keeping in primary care: a comparison of computerized, paper and hybrid systems. *BJGP* 2003; 53: 929–33.

4 Eve R. *PUNs and DENS. Discovering Learning Needs in General Practice*. Abingdon: Radcliffe Medical Press, 2003.

5 Rughani A. *The GP's Guide to Personal Development Plans*. Second edition. Abingdon: Radcliffe Medical Press, 2001.

6 Foster J, Jessop L and Dale J. Concerns and confidence of general practitioners in providing telephone consultations. *BJGP* 1999; 49: 111–13.

7 Hannis M D, Hazard R L, Rothschild M, Elnicki D M, Keyserling T C and DeVellis R F. Physician attitudes regarding telephone medicine. *Journal of General Internal Medicine* 1996; 11: 678–83.

8 Car J and Sheikh A. Telephone consultations. *BMJ* 2003; 326: 966–9.

Index

accessibility
  healthcare providers 208
  information 207, 211
accountability, GMC on 126
accreditation procedures
  and internet 208
  simulated patients 184–5
activity–passivity relationship model 38
adherence *see* compliance
advice calls 216, 234
advocates *see* patient advocates
agendas
  hidden 26, 227
  patients' 25–6, 27
aggression 97–9, 187–8
  author's reflections 99
alternative medicine 63
anger 97–9
  fear of 178
  signs of 97–8
  simulated patients 188, 190, 191, 192
  strategies 98
apology 98
assessment of communication 147–71
  author's reflections 169, 170
  blueprint 152–3
  clinical skills 147
  communication skills 147–8, 151
  content/process 161, 163–5
  design 151–4
    for high-stakes examinations 153
    validity/reliability 152, 153
  instruments 161–8
    checklists 163
    global marking 163
  knowledge 151, 152
  methods available 148
  model of medical expertise 151
  multi-source 161
  pass marks 153
  by patient feedback 159–60
  performance 156–61
    by medical officer 'sitting in' 158
    by simulated patients incognito 158–9
    by videotaping 157–8

by portfolios 160–1
rating 161–8
related issues 148–50
revalidation 148, 149
  criteria 169
  related issues 168–9
assessors 148
asylum seekers 118
  see also refugees
autonomy 39–40
  conflicting 47
availability bias 67

bad news
  breaking 92–6
    and doctor–patient relationship 93
    follow-up 93
    groundwork 93
    patient denial 94
    patient individuality 94, 96
    patient wishes 96
    prognoses 94
    SPIKES 94, 95
    strategies 94
    truthfulness 93
  definition 92
behavioural change
  motivational interviewing 96–7
  stages of change 96, 97
bias
  in published evidence 60
  in risk estimation 67
biomedical model 17–19
  definition 17
  disadvantages 19
biopsychosocial model 21
breaking bad news *see* bad news, breaking

case reliability 152
changes
  behavioural *see* behavioural change
  in doctor–patient relationship 126
  in general practice 105–24, 126
    affecting GPs 106
    author's reflections 121

consultation length 107–8
  due to consultation research 106–7
  in reality/perceptions 126–8
choice *see* doctor, choice of; informed
  choice; patient choice
chronic disease management 113
chronic multiple functional somatic
  symptoms (CMFS) 89
clinical competence *see* competence
clinical freedom 47
  constraints 47
Cochrane Collaboration on decision
  aids 69
Commonwealth Health Fund
  International Health Policy Survey
  of Sicker Adults 6, 49
communication
  across cultures 113–14
  errors 6
  methods 205–6
  patients with disabilities 92
communication skills
  assessment 146–7, 151
   related issues 148–50
  feelings, dealing with 134–5
  history of 128–9
  hospital doctors learning 121
  medical students learning 120
  and time constraints 139
  training
   controlled trial 131–4
   evaluation 132
   principles of 134
   in vocational training 5
community risk scale 68
community theatre 183
  see also North West Spanner
competence
  assessment 148–9
  definition 148
  definition/criteria 165
complexity theory 71
compliance 38
  and ISDM 48
complementary medicine 63
compression bias 67
computers *see* electronic record-keeping/
  communications

concordance 48
confidentiality 191, 192
  in advocacy 118
  ensuring 207, 208
  in training curriculum 9
conflict
  and anger 98
  of autonomy 47
  defensive strategies 86
  and EBM 63
  and empathy 85
  potential, examples of 82
  power 83
  strategies 83
conflict resolution 81–3, 98
consultation quality index 113
consultation skills
  in 20th century 128–9
  personal development plans 232–3
  see also assessment of communication
consultation template 223–35
  after consultation
   medical records 230–1
   personal development plans
   (PDPs) 232–3
    questions for 233
  before consultation 223
  choice of doctor 223–4
  consultation
   introductions 225–6
   opening remarks 226
   presentation/exploration of
   problems 226–7
   physical examination 227–8
   doctor/patient discussion
    agreement on plan 230
    health as whole 228–9
    nature/cause of problem(s) 228
    negotiation of management 229–
    30
   finishing off 230
   seeing nurse first 223–5
   telephone consultations 234–5
consultations
  content 20, 163–5
   assessment 161, 163
   influences on 108
  definition 15, 206

length
    changes in 107–8
    influences on 108
    minimum 223
    see also time constraints
methods
    movement between 27
    see also disease-centred approach;
    patient-centred approach;
    relationship-centred care
models 15–34
    early 15
process 20, 163–5
    assessment 161
consumerism 39
    vs patient partnership 46–7
content of consultation 20, 163
    assessment 161, 163
    content–process integration 20
    influences on 108
continuity of care 108–12, 223
    definition 109
    longitudinal *vs* personal continuity 109,
    110
    loss of personal continuity 110–11
    and medical history 111
control of consultation 26
    physician *vs* patient 38, 39
    see also power
criterion validity 152
culture 114
    cultural change in primary care 199
    cultural competency 113–16
        criticisms 115
        reductionist view 114
    cultural negotiation 116
    cultural preservation 115–16
    cultural repatterning 116

decision aids 69–70, 230
    definition 69
decision support 66
defensive overreactions 86
DENs 232
'dependent clingers' 88
descriptive explaining 79
difficult patients 88–91
    author's reflections 90, 100

consultation framework 89, 91
    and shared decision making 178
    simulated patients 191, 192
    work with SPs 190
Digital Divide 210
DIPEx database 127
disabilities, patients with 92
disease-centred approach 17–19
    doctor-centred nature 19
disease prevention 27, 229
doctor-centred approach 19
doctor, choice of 28, 223–4
doctor–computer communication 217–18
doctor–patient relationship
    changes over time 105
    in disease-centred approach 19
    legal issues 215
    models affecting management 38
doctor's educational needs (DEN) 232
'doorknob' comments 26
double-sided reflection 96
drug information, essential 66

e-patients 207
EBM *see* evidence-based medicine
education *see* training
educators
    author's personal journey 3–5
    GPs as 120–1
    and simulated patients 187
    working with patient movements 196–7
    see also patient teachers
electronic record-keeping/
    communications 205–19
    advantages/disadvantages 209
    augmenting consultations 216–17
    authentication 207–8
    author's reflections 218, 219
    Batman Belt Syndrome 208, 209
    confidentiality 208
    home visits 230–1
    individualised information/advice 217
    instant messaging 214
    integrated devices 209
    legal issues 214–16
    and non-verbal communication 212–13
    overload reduction strategies 210
    popularity 208

recording consultations 218
slow connections 210, 214
'store and forward' 214
validity of information 216
videoconferencing 212, 214
visibility of notes 212
voice recognition 217–18
email
   absence of non-verbal cues 212
   considerate use 211
   consultations 206
      standard protocol 207
emotional aspects of illness 27
empathy 77, 84–6
   angry patients 98
   criticism of 84
   definition 84
   empathic statements 85
   frequent attenders 89
   lack of 86
   in patient-centred approach 23
   in patient teachers 192
   pseudo-empathy 84
   two-stage process 85
   verbal/non-verbal 85
enhanced autonomy model 39
'entitled demanders' 88
equipoise, clinical 44
errors
   in published evidence 60
   in risk estimation 67
evidence-based medicine (EBM) 56–63
   definition 57
   deviation from 57–8
   evidence-related issues 59–61
      out-of-date information 61
      publication bias 60
      scepticism 59
   systematic reviews 60
   guidelines 62
   hierarchy of evidence 60
   searching skills 61–2
   shared decision making 62–3
   sources of evidence 61, 62
   steps for 57
examinations 153–4
   OSCE (objective structured clinical
   examination) 154–5

physical 17
simulated surgery 154–5
experiential learning 138–41
expert patients 3, 176–8
   author's reflections 199
experts
   definition 24
   on internet 207
   patients as 24, 63, 193
explaining 78–80
   adapting to patient 80
   checking patient understanding 79
   definition 78
   skills/strategies 80
   symptoms 87
   types of 78, 79

face validity 152
family doctor 17
five stages of change model 96, 97
frequent attenders 89–90
   author's reflections 90
   choice of doctor 224
   consultation framework 89, 91
   and internet information 211
Fresh Start 190, 198

General Medical Council see GMC
general practice
   changes
      affecting doctor–patient
      relationship 105–22
      affecting GPs 106
   core competencies 7–8
   training
      new curriculum 8–11
         on consultation context 8–9
         on consultation structure 10
         on professional attitudes in
         consultation 10–11
   WONCA definition 7–8
general practitioners (GPs)
   author's personal journey 2–3
   changes
      dislike of 105
      of role/demands on GP 106
   as educators 120–1, 197–8
   history 17

working with patients 197–8
　　GP's role/sense of identity 198–9
　　positive steps 198
GMC (General Medical Council)
　　on accountability 126
　　on good medical practice 7
　　revalidation 168–9
　　on undergraduate training 121
good medical practice 7–8
GP registrars 224
GPs *see* general practitioners
Groves's classification of 'hateful'
　　patients 88
guidance–cooperation relationship
　　model 38
guideline development 180

'hateful' patients, classification of 88
health promotion 225
　　and consultation time 107
　　discussion during consultation 27, 229
heartsink patients 88–91
hidden agendas 26, 227
history taking 17–18, 226
　　definition 17
　　frequent attenders 89
　　narrative medicine 24
　　reliability, improving 19
　　traditional 15
　　see also medical history
holism 110
honesty
　　about mistakes 98
　　breaking bad news 93

ICEE 22, 28
　　author's reflections 28
identity theft 207
influencing patient choices 42, 43, 82
information retention 65
information sharing 35–7
　　author's reflections 72
　　content 55–6
　　evidence/risks 55–73
　　frequent attenders/difficult patients 91
　　historical context 35–6
　　importance 37
　　legal issues 215–16

needs of patients 64
　　drug information, essential 66
　　specific questions 65
　　patient-centred approach 37–8
　　quantity/quality issues 63–6
　　reasons for failure 36–7
　　on risk 67
　　sources of information 64
　　suggested routine information 36
　　technical information 55, 56
　　underestimating patients' wishes 36
　　vs risk communication 40–1
　　vs shared decision making 41
information technology *see* electronic
　　record-keeping/communications
informed choice 39–40
informed consent 40–1
informed model consultation 39
informed shared decision making
　　(ISDM) 3, 41–4
　　author's reflections 49–50
　　compliance, improvement of 48
　　concordance, improvement of 48
　　doctor competencies 43
　　ensuring sharing of decisions 43
　　influencing patient choices 42, 43
　　junior doctors in 43
　　patients' views 44
Informed Shared Decision Making
　　Project 42
instant messaging 214
institutional racism 116
inter-case/inter-rater reliability 152
International Health Policy Survey of
　　Sicker Adults 6
internet 207, 209–10
　　augmenting consultations 216–17, 228
interns *see* pre-registration house officers
interpersonal skills 6
　　see also communication skills
interpreters, working with 116–17
interpretive explaining 79
ISDM *see* informed shared decision
　　making

jargon 37, 212
junior doctors 43, 80

knowledge 151, 152
'knowledge managers' 140

language problems 114, 116–17
learner-centred approach 130–1
  examples
    controlled trial 131–4
    experiential learning with simulated
    patients 138–40
    patients, preparing for 134–5
    work-based learning using
    video 136–8
learning
  confidence-building 187
  environment 141–2
  learning journey, patient's 196
  lifelong, and EBM 59
  patient voice in 175–201
  patients, changing role of 178–9
  from patients 179–80
    stages to success 180
  with patients 181–2
  peer support 136, 137
  work-based, with video 136–8
  see also training
legal issues 153
Leicester assessment package (LAP) 166
listening
  to learners 130–1
  new GPs 128
locum doctors 111, 224

management
  decisions
    decision support 66
    deviation from EBM 57–8
    disagreement 81
    factors affecting 58
    frequent attenders/difficult
    patients 91
    trial-of-one method 58, 59
  doctor–patient relationship models,
  effects of 38
'manipulative help-rejecters' 88
medical educators *see* educators
medical history 15, 16, 226
  components of 17–18
  frequent attenders/difficult patients 89, 91

patients' recall 18–19
  traditional 18
medical identity 176
medical records 230–1
  and electronic communications 215
  patient-held 111–12
medical students 120
  listening to patients 179
  responsibilities/attitudes 127–8
  role-play by 182–3
medically unexplained symptoms 89
Medicare-based practices 108
Mental Health in Higher Education
  (mhhe) group 197
migrants 118
Miller's pyramid 149
miscalibration bias 67
motivational interviewing 96–7
MRCGP
  College Membership examination 176
  fellowship examination 155–6
  statement of clinical competence 165
    elements of 164
multi-source assessment of
  communication 161
mutual participation 38

narrative medicine 24–5
negotiation 81–3
  definition 81
  of management 229–30
  in patient partnership 47
netiquette 205, 210
NLP (neurolinguistic programming) 99
non-verbal communication 85, 212–13
normalisation 45
North West Spanner 4, 129–30, 131
  see also Spanner Workshops
northern trainers' instrument for
  videotape assessment 165–6
nurse 224–5

objective structured clinical examination
  see OSCE
objective structured long examination
  record *see* OSLER
optimism–pessimism bias 67
OPTION (observing patient involvement)

162, 166–7
options
  discussion of
    incomplete information 56
    influencing patient choices 42, 43, 82
  effective *vs* preference sensitive 66
OSCE (objective structured clinical
  examination) 154–5, 184
OSLER (objective structured long
  examination record) 154
Oxbridge Rating Scale 132, 133

paternalism 16–17, 19, 35
  breaking bad news 93
  persisting 46
  and uncertainty 70
patient advocates 118
patient agendas *see* agendas, patients'
patient-centred approach 20–1
  assessment 162
  attributes required 23
  author's reflections 30
  breaking bad news 93
  conflict 82–3
  doctors' reactions 27
  evidence of usefulness 23–4
  factors hindering adoption 29
  information sharing 37–8
  and language barriers 117
  negotiation/conflict resolution 81
  patients' reactions 27, 28
  related issues 26–8
patient-centred clinical method 21–2, 37
patient choice 126
patient enablement instrument (PAI) 167–8
patient-held records 111–12
patient instructors 183
patient involvement 20–1
  emergent issues 182
  history 16
  practice development 179–80
  role in doctors' learning 178–9
  structure/method establishment 196–7
  training/education 181–2
  see also patient voice
patient-led NHS, development of 197
patient partnership 46
  author's reflection 49

erosion of 16–17
  vs consumerism 46–7
patient perspective 128–9
  eliciting 129–30
patient profile changes 106
patient self-management 80–1, 177
patient teachers 5, 176–8, 192
Patients as Teachers group 193, 195
patient voice 4, 5, 129–30
  definition 176
  in doctors' learning 175–201
  eliciting authentic voices 195–7
  as evaluation tool 23
  obstacles to hearing, overcoming 197
  shaping/validating learning
  materials 193
  and simulated patients 182
    aggression 187–8
    background 182–4
    development for patient roles 188
    effectiveness, steps to 184–5
    evaluating SP work 184–5
    examples
      assumptions/stereotypes,
      overcoming 190–2
      end-of-life decision making 194–5
      shaping/validating learning 193–4
    facilitation 186–7
    feedback 189–90
    preparing a role 188–9
    problems using SPs 177
    safety 187–8
  in SP accreditation 184–5
  see also patient involvement
patients
  as fellow workers 178
  role in doctors' learning 178–9
  as teachers *see* patient teachers
Patients as Teachers group 193, 195
Patient's Charter 126
patient's unmet needs (PUN) 232
peer assessment questionnaire 162
perceptions, changing 126–8
performance
  components 149–50
  definition 148
Personal and Professional Development
  (PPD) 135

personal care 109, 110
personal development plans (PDPs) 232–3
personal digital assistants (PDAs) 212
pervasive technology 210–12
physical examination, historical
  importance of 17
*Policy Paper on Information Technology
  and Rural Health* 213
portfolios
  assessment of communication by 161
  definition 160
power
  in conflicts 83
  dimensions 39–40
  in doctor–patient relationship 126–7
practice nurse 225
pre-registration house officers (PRHOs) 120
prejudice 116, 117
Preparing for Patients 134–5
Preparing Professionals for Participation
  with the Public 180
presenting complaints 87, 227
  and hidden agendas 26
  resolved 25–6
  see also symptoms
primary care
  cultural change 199
history 17
  roles/relationships, proposed changes
    in 198–9
process of consultation 20, 163
  assessment 161, 163
  content–process integration 20
pseudo-empathy 84
psychological aspects
  attributing symptoms to 90
  of illness 21
psychosocial issues 137
  and consultation time 107
  risk, reaction to 69
publication bias 60
PUNs 232

Quality and Outcomes Framework
  (QoF) 113
quality of care 112–13
  measurement 113

racism 116
RCGP (Royal College of General
  Practitioners)
  on good medical practice 7
  membership examination 147
  simulated consultations 182
  see also MRCGP
realities, changing 126–8
reason-giving explaining 79
'reasonable person' standard 40
recording consultations 218, 230
records *see* medical history
referral 230
reflection, double-sided 96
refugees 118, 119, 136
relationship-centred care 22–3
  enhanced autonomy model 39
reliability of assessment 152, 153
resourceful patients 127
respect 184, 192
retention of information 65
revalidation of assessment 148, 149
  criteria 169
  related issues 168–9
risk
  communication 66–9
    author's reflection 72
    influences on response 67
    informed consent as 40
    language 68
    risk scales 68–9
  definition 66
  errors in estimation 67
role-play 4, 129–30, 182–3
Royal College of General Practitioners
  (RCGP) *see* RCGP
Royal College of Physicians 182
Royal College of Surgeons 182
rural healthcare 210, 213

safety
  and angry patients 98–9
  simulated patients 187, 192
'self-destructive deniers' 88
self-management
  and explanation 80–1
  in future 177
shared decision making 24, 26, 35–50

assessment 162
author's reflections 49
breaking bad news 93
characteristics 42
to do nothing 44–5
EBM-based decisions 62–3
frequent attenders/difficult patients 91
informed *see* informed shared decision
making
lack of 49
and language barriers 117
medical students learning 120
negotiation/conflict resolution 81
objections to 45–6
recording discussions 231
schematic diagram 50
'wait and see' scenario 44
shared information *see* information
sharing
shared model *see* informed shared
decision making
shared narrative 25
shared protocols and continuity of
care 111
shared understanding 37–8
simulated patients (SPs) 3, 5, 177
accreditation procedures 184–5
and aggression 187
angry/difficult patients 188, 190, 191, 192
in controlled trial 132
debriefing structure 187
examples
assumptions/stereotypes,
overcoming 190–2
end-of-life decision making 194–5
manipulative/criminal behaviour,
coping with 188–9
shaping/validating learning
materials 193–4
experiential learning 138–40
feedback
in/out of role 189–90
structure 185–7
and patient voice 182
aggression 187–8
background 182–4
development for patient roles 188
effectiveness, steps to 184–5

evaluating SP work 184–5
facilitation 185–7
feedback 189–90
preparing a role 188–9
problems using SPs 177
safety 187–8
in performance assessment 159
preparation 184–5
recruitment/selection 185
safety 187–8, 192
social aspects of illness 19, 21, 22, 27
psychosocial issues 69, 107, 137
social deprivation 118
social justice 118–19
spam 205, 211
Spanner Workshops 131, 132, 138
see also North West Spanner
speech impairment 92
SPIKES 94, 95
SPs *see* simulated patients
standards 7–8
students *see* medical students
symptoms
chronic multiple functional somatic
(CMFS) 89
dealing with 86–8
definition 86
explanation of 87
medically unexplained 89
see also presenting complaints

team working 111–12, 161
technology, pervasive 210–12
telehealth 212–13
legal issues 214–16
limitations 213
telephone consultations 216–17, 234–5
content/process 235
protocol 234
quality assessmentv234
telephone return calls 216, 234
template for consultation *see* consultation
template
theatre company involvement 4, 129–30
see also North West Spanner; Spanner
Workshops
time constraints
and communication skills 139

consultation length, changes in 107–8
patient-centred approach 27, 29, 30
shared decision making 45
TLAs (three letter acronyms) 205, 212
training 129–30
  communication skills 5
    controlled trial 131–4
    evaluation 132
    involving patients 136–7
    principles of 134
    in vocational training 5
  general practice 131
  learner-centred approach 130–1
    examples 131–40
  learners in difficulty 138
  learning environment 141–2
  new curriculum 8–11
  patient involvement 181–2
  Personal and Professional Development
  (PPD) 135
  personal development plans 232
  reflective learning 136, 137, 141
  role-play 4, 129–30
  undergraduate, GMC on 121
  see also educators; learning
truthfulness see honesty

uncertainty
  doctors coping with 70–1
  in early consultation 71
  and overprescription 87–8
  patients coping with 71–2
understanding
  checking, after explaining 79
  patients with disabilities 92
  shared 37–8

validity
  of assessment 152, 153
  of electronic information 216
verbal/non-verbal communication 85,
  212–13
videoconferencing 214
  absence of non-verbal cues 212
videotaping
  assessment of tapes 165–6
  for skill assessment 149, 156, 157, 158
  for skill development 2, 3, 149

simulated patients in 194–5
  for work-based learning 136–8
violence see aggression
voice recognition technology 217–18

walk-in centres 112
websites 207
'Where's the Patient Voice in Health
  Professional Education?' 181
WONCA (World Organization of Family
  Doctors)
    definition of general practice 7–8
    Policy Paper on Information
    Technology and Rural Health 213
work-based learning
  with patient perspective 140–1
  using video 136–8
Working for Patients 126
World Health Organization on roles/
  relationships in primary care 198–9